Cell-based Therapies in Orthopedics

Guest Editors

MATTHEW C. STEWART, BVSc,
MVetClinStud, PhD
ALLISON A. STEWART, DVM, MS

VETERINARY CLINICS OF NORTH AMERICA: EQUINE PRACTICE

www.vetequine.theclinics.com

Consulting Editor
ANTHONY SIMON TURNER, BVSc, MS

August 2011 • Volume 27 • Number 2

SAUNDERS an imprint of ELSEVIER, Inc.

W.B. SAUNDERS COMPANY
A Division of Elsevier Inc.

1600 John F. Kennedy Boulevard ● Suite 1800 ● Philadelphia, Pennsylvania 19103

http://www.vetequine.theclinics.com

VETERINARY CLINICS OF NORTH AMERICA: EQUINE PRACTICE Volume 27, Number 2

August 2011 ISSN 0749-0739, ISBN-13: 978-1-4557-0519-1

Editor: John Vassallo; j.vassallo@elsevier.com

Veterinary Clinics of North America: Equine Practice (ISSN 0749-0739) is published in April, August, and December by Elsevier Inc., 360 Park Avenue South, New York, NY 10010-1710. Business and Editorial Offices: 1600 John F. Kennedy Blvd., Suite 1800, Philadelphia, PA 19103-2899. Subscription prices are $238.00 per year (domestic individuals), $373.00 per year (domestic institutions), $117.00 per year (domestic students/residents), $277.00 per year (Canadian individuals), $466.00 per year (Canadian institutions), $320.00 per year (international individuals), $466.00 per year (international institutions), and $159.00 per year (international and Canadian students/residents). To receive student/resident rate, orders must be accompanied by name of affiliated institution, date of term, and the signature of program/residency coordinator on institution letterhead. Orders will be billed at individual rate until proof of status is received. Foreign air speed delivery is included in all *Clinics* subscription prices. All prices are subject to change without notice. **POSTMASTER:** Send address changes to *Veterinary Clinics of North America: Equine Practice*, 3251 Riverport Lane, Maryland Heights, MO 63043. Customer Service (orders, claims, online, change of address): Elsevier Health Sciences Division, Subscription Customer Service, 3251 Riverport Lane, Maryland Heights, MO 63043. Tel: 1-800-654-2452 (U.S. and Canada); 314-447-8871 (outside U.S. and Canada). Fax: 314-447-8029. E-mail: journalscustomer service-usa@elsevier.com (for print support); E-mail: journalsonlinesupport-usa@elsevier (for online support).

Reprints. For copies of 100 or more of articles in this publication, please contact the Commercial Reprints Department, Elsevier Inc., 360 Park Avenue South, New York, NY 10010-1710. Tel.: 212-633-3812; Fax: 212-462-1935; E-mail: reprints@elsevier.com.

Veterinary Clinics of North America: Equine Practice is covered in *MEDLINE/PubMed (Index Medicus), Excerpta Medica, Current Contents/Agriculture, Biology and Environmental Sciences, and ISI.*

Printed and bound by CPI Group (UK) Ltd, Croydon, CR0 4YY

Transferred to Digital Print 2011

Contributors

CONSULTING EDITOR

ANTHONY SIMON TURNER, BVSc, MS
Diplomate, American College of Veterinary Surgeons; Professor, Department of Clinical Sciences, College of Veterinary Medicine and Biomedical Sciences, Colorado State University, Fort Collins, Colorado

GUEST EDITORS

MATTHEW C. STEWART, BVSc (Hons 1), MVetClinStud, PhD
Fellow of the Australian College of Veterinary Scientists (Equine Surgery); Associate Professor of Equine Surgery, Director of Graduate Studies and Research, Department of Veterinary Clinical Medicine, College of Veterinary Medicine, University of Illinois, Urbana, Illinois

ALLISON A. STEWART, DVM, MS
Diplomate, American College of Veterinary Surgeons; Associate Professor of Equine Surgery, Department of Veterinary Clinical Medicine, College of Veterinary Medicine, University of Illinois, Urbana, Illinois

AUTHORS

A.G.L. ALVES, DVM, MS, PhD
Professor, Department of Veterinary Surgery and Anesthesiology, School of Veterinary Medicine and Animal Science, São Paulo State University, Botucatu, São Paulo, Brazil

DORI L. BORJESSON, DVM, PhD
Diplomate, American College of Veterinary Pathologists; Associate Professor, Department of Pathology, Microbiology and Immunology, School of Veterinary Medicine, University of California, Davis, California

PETER D. CLEGG, MA, Vet MB, PhD
Diplomate, European College of Veterinary Surgeons; Professor of Equine Surgery, Department of Musculoskeletal Biology, Faculty of Health and Life Sciences, University of Liverpool, Neston, Cheshire, United Kingdom

JAY DUDHIA, PhD
Department of Veterinary Clinical Sciences, The Royal Veterinary College, University of London, Hatfield, Hertfordshire, United Kingdom

LISA A. FORTIER, DVM, PhD
Diplomate, American College of Veterinary Surgeons; Associate Professor, Department of Clinical Sciences, Veterinary Medical Center, College of Veterinary Medicine, Cornell University, Ithaca, New York

DAVID D. FRISBIE, DVM, PhD
Diplomate, American College of Veterinary Surgeons; Diplomate, American College of Veterinary Sports Medicine and Rehabilitation; Associate Professor, Equine Orthopaedic Research Center, Department of Clinical Sciences, College of Veterinary Medicine and Biological Sciences; Molecular, Cellular and Tissue Engineering, Department of Mechanical Engineering, School of Biomedical Engineering, Colorado State University, Fort Collins, Colorado

ALLEN E. GOODSHIP, BVSc, PhD, MRCVS
Professor, Institute of Orthopaedics and Musculoskeletal Science, University College London, Royal National Orthopaedic Hospital, Stanmore, Middlesex, United Kingdom

SANTIAGO D. GUTIERREZ-NIBEYRO, DVM, MS
Diplomate, American College of Veterinary Surgeons; Clinical Assistant Professor of Equine Surgery, Department of Clinical Veterinary Medicine, College of Veterinary Medicine, University of Illinois, Champaign-Urbana, Illinois

CATHERINE H. HACKETT, DVM, PhD
Diplomate, American College of Veterinary Surgeons; Post Doctoral Fellow, Department of Clinical Sciences, Veterinary Medical Center, College of Veterinary Medicine, Cornell University, Ithaca, New York

YOSHINORI KASASHIMA, DVM, PhD
Clinical Science and Pathology Division, Equine Research Institute, Japan Racing Association, Utsunomiya, Tochigi, Japan

PETER I. MILNER, BVetMed, BSc(Hons), PhD, CertES(Orth), MRCVS
Lecturer in Equine Orthopaedics, Department of Musculoskeletal Biology, Faculty of Health and Life Sciences, University of Liverpool, Neston, Cheshire, United Kingdom

KARL M. NOBERT, ESQ
Food and Drug Regulatory Attorney, K&L Gates LLP, Washington, DC

JOHN F. PERONI, DVM, MS
Diplomate, American College of Veterinary Surgeons; Associate Professor of Large Animal Surgery, Department of Large Animal Medicine, College of Veterinary Medicine, University of Georgia, Athens, Georgia

GINA L. PINCHBECK, BVSc, PhD
Diplomate, European College of Veterinary Public Health; Senior Lecturer in Epidemiology, Department of Epidemiology, Faculty of Health and Life Sciences, University of Liverpool, Neston, Cheshire, United Kingdom

ROGER K.W. SMITH, MA, VetMB, PhD, DEO, DipECVS, MRCVS
Professor, Department of Veterinary Clinical Sciences, The Royal Veterinary College, University of London, Hatfield, Hertfordshire, United Kingdom

ALLISON A. STEWART, DVM, MS
Diplomate, American College of Veterinary Surgeons; Associate Professor of Equine Surgery, Department of Veterinary Clinical Medicine, College of Veterinary Medicine, University of Illinois, Urbana, Illinois

MATTHEW C. STEWART, BVSc (Hons 1), MVetClinStud, PhD
Fellow of the Australian College of Veterinary Scientists (Equine Surgery); Associate Professor of Equine Surgery, Director of Graduate Studies and Research, Department of Veterinary Clinical Medicine, College of Veterinary Medicine, University of Illinois, Urbana, Illinois

SARAH E. TAYLOR, BVM&S, MSc, PhD, Cert ES(Orth), MRCVS
Diplomate, European College of Veterinary Surgeons; Senior Lecturer in Equine
Orthopaedic Surgery, Department of Veterinary Clinical Sciences, University of
Edinburgh, Dick Vet Equine Hospital, Easter Bush Vet Centre, Roslin, Midlothian,
United Kingdom

JAMIE TEXTOR, DVM
Diplomate, American College of Veterinary Surgeons; PhD Candidate, Tablin Laboratory,
Department of Pathology, Microbiology and Immunology, College of Veterinary Medicine,
University of California Davis, Davis, California

Contents

The field of regenerative medicine research is rapidly expanding. One area of interest to equine researchers is the possibility of isolating or generating pluripotent cells, capable of producing differentiated cell types derived from all 3 primary germ layers. Reports of equine embryonic stem-like (ES) cell isolation can be found in the literature. Other groups are working to produce equine-induced pluripotent stem (iPS) cells. This article summarizes the essential features needed to characterize a cell type as pluripotent, specific challenges in using the horse as a model organism for pluripotent cell generation, and current and upcoming clinical trials using ES/iPS cells.

This article provides an overview of mesenchymal stem cell (MSC) biology. In the first section, the characteristics that are routinely used to define MSCs—adherence, proliferation, multi-lineage potential, and "cluster of differentiation" marker profiles—are discussed. In the second section, the major tissues and body fluids that are used as sources for equine MSCs are presented, along with the comparative biologic activities of MSCs from specific locations. Finally, the current understanding of the mechanisms by which MSCs influence repair and regeneration are discussed, with an emphasis on the clinical importance of MSC trophic activities.

Mesenchymal stromal cells (MSC) are derived from adult mesenchymal tissues and have the ability to undergo differentiation into bone, cartilage, and fat, and have therefore attracted great interest in regenerative medicine. Many isolation and culture methods have been described, making comparison between laboratories and quality-control protocols difficult. A uniform protocol to characterize equine MSC has recently been proposed, aiming to introduce consistency across the equine stem cell research field. This article reviews the published techniques for collection and propagation of equine MSC, focusing on bone marrow–derived and adipose-derived cells.

Autologous biologic therapies such as platelet-rich plasma and autologous conditioned serum are in widespread clinical use to treat musculoskeletal pathology in horses. These substances exert a therapeutic effect through the provision of either anabolic or anti-catabolic factors, or a combination of both. This article discusses the history, experimental and clinical literature, and currently accepted preparation and usage strategies for both platelet-rich plasma and autologous conditioned serum.

Several cell-based therapeutic options to treat musculoskeletal injuries in horses are commercially available. The current literature supports the use of cell-based therapies to treat equine musculoskeletal injuries. Researchers continue to search for more effective cell-based therapies to provide practitioners with optimal treatment tools for musculoskeletal injuries in horses. Cell-based therapies require specialized facilities and technical competencies that might not be available or economically justifiable in many private practices. This review provides a summary of current commercially available cell-based therapeutic products for equine applications, their similarities and differences, and current objective data relating to their clinical efficacy.

Evidence-based medicine (EBM) refers to the conscientious, explicit, and judicious use of current best evidence from research for the care of an individual patient. Central to the adoption of EBM is both producing and identifying the best possible evidence for a particular intervention or therapy. This article identifies and reviews the approaches to producing and identifying the best possible evidence that is necessary for the full acceptance of stem cell therapies in the horse and reviews the approaches that will allow future clinical studies in stem cell therapies to provide the best evidence for determining efficacy.

This article provides an overview of the US Food and Drug Administration's current and potential regulation of veterinary regenerative medicine and the various products used in the practice. This article also discusses several of the potential enforcement risks associated with the commercialization of such therapies and products and offers the reader strategies for mitigating those risks. Finally, the article concludes with a review of an important and ongoing court battle that focuses on the marketing and promotion of cellular-based therapies for humans that could have a significant impact on the regulation of both human and veterinary products.

This article focuses on current issues facing cell-based therapies in equine practice and future studies validating the use of stem cells and related biologic therapies for the treatment of musculoskeletal conditions in the horse. Issues raised include the characterization and use of tissue- and anatomic location–specific mesenchymal stem cell (MSC) sources, the putative advantages and feasibility of allogeneic embryonic stem cell and

MSC products, the technical advantages and performance of cell-based biologic agents that do not require extensive *ex vivo* manipulation, the regulation of MSC homing, potential nonorthopaedic stem cell applications, and the logistics required to demonstrate cell-based therapy efficacy in horses.

THE CLINICS ARE NOW AVAILABLE ONLINE!

Access your subscription at:
www.theclinics.com

Preface

Cell-based Therapies in Orthopedics

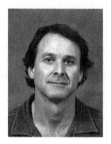 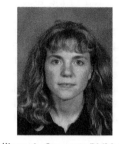

Matthew C. Stewart, BVSc,   Allison A. Stewart, DVM, MS
MVetClinStud, PhD
Guest Editors

Cell-based therapies are the current "hot topic" in both the biomedical and veterinary communities. Research and development in this field has been remarkable in recent years, driven by the promise of true regenerative healing and effective treatments for recalcitrant degenerative conditions.

The equine veterinary profession, in many respects, leads the field in cell-based therapies for musculoskeletal and orthopedic conditions, motivated by the limitations of our current treatments and the high rates of failure and recurrence for conditions such as long bone fracture, flexor tendinitis, and osteoarthritis. Biologically based therapies are particularly attractive for use in performance horses because, at least so far, their administration is not subject to any regulatory withholding period before competition. Accepting the much referred to potential of stem cells and other cell-based approaches, it is clear that the current widespread treatment of horses with stem cell formulations, aspirates, and tissue concentrates is not yet backed by substantive and compelling data. Cell-based therapy is very much a work in progress at this stage. The material in this volume provides a comprehensive overview of cell-based therapies for the treatment of musculoskeletal and orthopedic conditions in the horse and presents the experimental and clinical studies that do (and do not) support cell-based therapy in specific clinical conditions.

The first 4 articles of this edition are focused on the primary sources of cell-based therapies: embryonic stem cells and induced pluripotent cells (Hackett and Fortier), mesenchymal stem cells (chapters by Stewart, and Stewart, and by Taylor and Clegg), and platelet-rich plasma cells and interleukin 1 receptor antagonist protein (Textor). The next group of articles covers cell-based therapies for specific equine musculoskeletal conditions, focusing on current cell-based therapies for bone repair (Milner, Clegg, and Stewart), the treatment of tendon injuries (Alves and colleagues), joint diseases

Vet Clin Equine 27 (2011) xiii–xiv
doi:10.1016/j.cveq.2011.07.002
0749-0739/11/$ – see front matter © 2011 Elsevier Inc. All rights reserved.

(Frisbie and Stewart), and the application of stem cells as immunomodulatory agents (Peroni and Borjesson). The rapidly increasing number of commercial resources for cell-based therapies in equine practice is covered in the article by Gutierrez-Nibeyro. The articles by Clegg and Pinchbeck and also by Nobert, although not primarily clinical in their content, are perhaps the most important for the future development of cell-based therapies in equine practice. The existing evidence for clinical efficacy of cell-based therapies in horses is presented in the article by Clegg and Pinchbeck; to summarize, there is little high-quality data to support these therapies at this time. In the Nobert article, the legal aspects of cell-based therapy use in horses are covered in detail, drawing heavily on the regulatory practices that are currently applied to biological treatments in human medicine. The implications of more-stringent Food and Drug Administration regulation of veterinary use of cell-based and biological therapies are concerning, in light of the logistics and costs associated with any demonstration of clinical efficacy. The final article presents a brief overview of current issues relating to cell-based therapies in equine practice and future challenges for the equine veterinary profession.

We would like to thank all the authors who contributed to this issue, both for the outstanding coverage of this complex and rapidly expanding field and for their willingness to present their personal experience with the use of, and outcomes from, cell-based therapies in their equine patients. We are also thankful to Dr Simon Turner for giving us the opportunity to be involved in this VCNA edition and to John Vassallo for his guidance, endless patience, and the strength to resist treating us as we undoubtedly deserved as deadline after deadline passed by!

Matthew C. Stewart, BVSc, MVetClinStud, PhD
Allison A. Stewart, DVM, MS
Department of Veterinary Clinical Medicine
College of Veterinary Medicine
University of Illinois
1008 West Hazelwood Drive
Urbana, IL 61802, USA

E-mail addresses:
matt1@illinois.edu (M.C. Stewart)
aaw@illinois.edu (A.A. Stewart)

Embryonic Stem Cells and iPS Cells: Sources and Characteristics

Catherine H. Hackett, DVM, PhD, Lisa A. Fortier, DVM, PhD*

KEYWORDS

- Embryonic stem cell • Induced pluripotent stem cell
- Differentiation • Tissue regeneration

By definition, embryonic stem (ES) cells are pluripotent, meaning they can form tissues from all 3 primary germ layers (ectoderm, endoderm, and mesoderm) of the embryo. This differs from totipotency in that pluripotent ES cells cannot form placental tissues, and therefore ES cells cannot form a viable embryo without contributions from other cell types. The mammalian embryo is totipotent up to the 16-cell stage, after which the cells of the morula begin to differentiate to defined fates. Multipotency defines cells that have the potential to form 2 or more differentiated tissues, but not necessarily form multiple germ layers.

Induced pluripotent stem (iPS) cells are somatic cells that have been reprogrammed to behave like an ES cell by artificially turning on expression of specific pluripotency genes. This reprogramming can be achieved using a number of techniques with varying efficiencies. Many iPS cell lines share gene expression patterns and epigenetic traits of ES cells; however, the exact relationship between ES and iPS cells is still poorly understood. Numerous differences have been identified between ES and iPS cells that may have significant impact on the future clinical use of each cell type. The methods to derive ES and iPS cell lines are distinct from each other and will be discussed separately. In contrast, the methods used to characterize these cell types are similar and will be discussed together.

ES CELLS
Tissue Sources and Isolation

ES cells are derived from the inner cell mass of the blastocyst stage embryo. In people, this stage occurs at 5 to 6 days after fertilization,[1] and the mouse at 3 to 4 days after fertilization.[2] There have been several reports describing the generation of ES-like

The authors have nothing to disclose.
Department of Clinical Sciences, Box 32, Veterinary Medical Center, College of Veterinary Medicine, Cornell University, Ithaca, NY 14853, USA
* Corresponding author.
E-mail address: laf4@cornell.edu

cells from horses.[3–7] Embryo collection for equine ES cell isolation has been reported to range from 6 to 8 days after fertilization.[4,6,7] During this time period, the harvested equine embryo is in a blastocyst or an expanded blastocyst stage. To date, no reported equine ES cell lines have been proven to be pluripotent in any in vivo assay. The absence of any data verifying in vivo pluripotency prevents definitive classification of these cells as true ES cell lines.[8]

Two methods have been used to isolate the inner cell mass of the blastocyst for ES cell isolation. Across species, the most frequently used method is microsurgery. This procedure involves mechanical dissection under microscopic guidance and manual separation of the inner cell mass from trophoblastic lineage cells. The second method involves immunodissection using an antibody that targets trophoblast lineage cells of the blastocyst. Complement is added to the antibody-labeled blastocyst, leading to destruction of trophoblastic lineage cells while the inner cell mass remains unharmed. Both microsurgical dissection and immunosurgical dissection have been described for isolation of the equine inner cell mass.[4,6,7]

ES Cell Advantages

For clinical application, a fully validated ES cell product would have a number of advantages over currently available cell-based products. First, ES cells have the potential to replicate indefinitely under defined conditions without differentiation, making an off-the-shelf preparation possible. Next, ES cells are able to form many committed cell types for regenerative tissue repair when differentiated before implantation. Another significant advantage is that there is minimal genetic manipulation of ES cells, and there is a consequently decreased risk of aberrant tumor formation compared with iPS cell lines. ES cells have potential value in the treatment of genetic diseases through therapeutic cloning applications. ES cells have been used extensively in the production of transgenic mice, demonstrating proof of principle of their potential value with genetic manipulation.

ES Cell Disadvantages

Despite the tremendous potential ES cells hold for clinical benefit, several disadvantages need to be addressed. Routinely used methods for inner cell mass isolation necessitate destruction of an embryo, leading to ethical concerns across species, but especially in human ES cell research. Another concern for clinical application of ES cells is the potential for allogenic immunogenicity. Since ES cells are somewhat immunoprivileged, this may be less of a concern in therapeutic uses. One important disadvantage is the need for specific, complicated culture conditions to propagate and maintain ES cell lines in an undifferentiated state and the requirement for frequent monitoring of cultured cells for changes in genomic state to assure phenotypic stability.[9] Additionally, there is a risk for tumor formation if ES cells are not fully directed into a differentiated cell type before surgical implantation. For therapeutic applications in people, another major concern is the use of nonhuman materials such as fetal bovine serum and mouse feeder cells to derive ES cells. An added problem to address is that the genetic background of the blastocyst plays an important role in the efficiency of deriving ES cell lines, as has been clearly demonstrated in the mouse.[10] Horses have much more genetic variability than typical inbred mouse strains; therefore equine ES cell line generation may be complicated by their inconsistent genetic background. Horses have the additional disadvantages of low embryo numbers to harvest during blastocyst collection and lack of optimal culture conditions to promote equine ES cell expansion without differentiation.

iPS CELLS
Tissue Sources, Isolation, and Induction

Any nucleated somatic cell in the body can theoretically be reprogrammed using iPS techniques. Many human and murine studies have used skin cells and fibroblasts for the initial adult cell source. Adult neural stem cells have been reported as the initial cell type in cellular reprogramming studies.[11] Recently, a group has described the reprogramming of murine bone marrow mononuclear cells with higher efficiency than mouse embryonic fibroblasts.[12]

Numerous methods have been used to induce the reprogramming of non-ES cells. The initial techniques described used retroviral or lentiviral transfections to induce expression of oncogenes into the candidate cell following viral incorporation into the host cell's genome.[13–15] Later work demonstrated that adenoviral vectors could be used that would avoid viral incorporation into the host genome.[16] Use of adenoviral vectors may be a safer alternative compared with retroviral or lentiviral vectors; however, the gene expression induced by adenoviral vectors is not maintained long term in transduced cells, limiting their pluripotent longevity. Expression plasmids alone have been used to induce pluripotency genes in target cells, but generation of iPS colonies is extremely inefficient using this method. Concern about the use of viral vectors has led other groups to attempt reprogramming of human fibroblasts using direct delivery of proteins into cells, again with poor efficiency.[17] Recently, a significant advance was described using the introduction of modified mRNA to reprogram adult cells.[18] This group went on to demonstrate proof of concept that induced cells can be directed to a specific lineage using the modified RNA technique. The modified RNA reprogramming method may prove to be the safest and most efficient strategy to reprogram adult cells and promote subsequent differentiation into the desired cell product for eventual therapeutic use.

Although several groups are currently working to develop equine iPS cell lines, only 1 group has published a report of definitive iPS production in the horse.[19] The field of cellular reprogramming is changing rapidly, and adaptation of techniques developed for other species will likely prove useful to enhance the induction of equine cells to a pluripotent state in the near future. For example, a recent report describes surgical implantation of chemically induced putative ES-like cells in an equine model of superficial digital flexor tendonitis, leading to improved histologic repair in the ES-like cell treated versus control lesions.[20]

iPS Cell Advantages

iPS cells should be less prone to immunorejection, since they can be patient-derived or major histocompatibility complex (MHC) class 1-matched for compatibility. Production of iPS cell lines also avoids the ethical controversy of embryo destruction associated with ES cell generation. In the horse, abundant donor tissues (eg, dermal fibroblasts isolated from skin biopsies) are available to provide ample initial adult cells for reprogramming.

iPS Cell Disadvantages

The use of viral vectors (especially retroviruses or lentiviruses that randomly incorporate into the host genome) for iPS colony generation increases the risk of tumor formation and leads to concern for transplantation of reprogrammed cells in clinical trials. Overall, an increased risk of tumor formation has been demonstrated in human iPS cells compared with ES cells.[21] iPS cells can also show dramatic variability in the completeness of reprogramming and require extensive screening to select the most

ES-like cells. Similar to cultured ES cells, cultured iPS cells need to be frequently monitored for genomic abnormalities to ensure clinical safety.[9]

FACTORS TO INDUCE OR DEFINE PLURIPOTENCY

Many different combinations of pluripotency factors have been described for defining pluripotency or reprogramming cells with varying efficiencies in iPS cell colony generation or ES/iPS cell validation. All of the pluripotency induction genes have been previously linked to cancer, suggesting a connection between oncogenic transformation and pluripotency. The gene and protein expression pattern of fully reprogrammed cells and ES cells varies slightly by species; however, both types of cells must express the genes POU5F1, SOX2, NANOG, and TERT. ES/iPS cells also require a high level of telomerase activity to sustain self-renewal and proliferation. The following factors have been reported to contribute to iPS generation and are useful to evaluate ES and iPS pluripotency.

Octamer-binding protein (Oct 3/4) has been used in nearly all cellular reprogramming strategies. It is a homeodomain transcription factor encoded by the gene POU5F1. A precise quantity of Oct 3/4 protein is needed to control cellular differentiation or maintenance of pluripotency. An excess of Oct 3/4 leads to spontaneous differentiation of ES cells into either primitive endoderm or mesoderm, while a deficiency in protein expression leads to a trophoectoderm phenotype.[22] One study has demonstrated POU5F1gene transfection can be used as a single factor (although with extremely low efficiency) to reprogram adult neural stem cells.[23] Oct 3/4 is considered to be one of the master regulators of pluripotency in conjunction with Sox2 and Nanog.

Sex-determining region Y-box 2 (Sox2) is a less-specific transcription factor that plays a role in pluripotency induction and other differentiation processes. For example, Sox2 is expressed in large quantities in developing and adult neural tissue[24] and plays an important role in the regulation of Oct 3/4 expression.[25] The Sox2 and Oct 3/4 proteins form a heterodimer that binds DNA and regulates the expression of many other genes involved in embryonic development.

Nanog is a transcription factor important to the maintenance of undifferentiated ES cells and is a key gene in the regulation of pluripotency.[26] Although not absolutely required as a transduction factor, Nanog expression has been shown to be upregulated in iPS cells and is a good marker of cellular reprogramming.[27] Overexpression of Nanog permits pluripotent self-renewal in human ES cells without the use of feeder cells or specialized media supplements.[28] In addition, it has been shown that the tumor suppressor p53 binds to the promoter of Nanog, resulting in down-regulation of gene expression following DNA damage, and leading to differentiation of ES cells.[29]

c-Myc is a proto-oncogene commonly linked to neoplastic transformation. In addition to functioning as a transcription factor, c-Myc and the other Myc family members also play a role in modification of chromatin structure through recruitment of histone acetyltransferases.[30] Although c-Myc improves the efficiency of iPS cell generation, about 20% of chimeric mice produced from c-Myc induced iPS cells developed cancer.[13] Ultimately, iPS production strategies to be used clinically should avoid the use of Myc family members as reprogramming factors.

Kruppel-like factor 4 (Klf4) is a member of a family of transcription factors with important roles in cell proliferation, differentiation, and survival. It was one of the key factors used by Yamanaka's group in the first description of murine iPS generation.[13] Subsequently, other Klf family members have been used to generate iPS cells. In contrast, other research groups have demonstrated human iPS cells can be generated without addition of a Klf family member.[14]

Lin28 serves as an mRNA-binding protein and enhances the efficiency of iPS cell generation.[14] Its main function is to enhance the translation of specific proteins, leading to more efficient protein synthesis. Lin28 is also expressed during fetal liver development and in cells undergoing muscle or neural differentiation and is therefore not a specific marker of pluripotency.

CULTURE OF ES/iPS CELLS

Propagation of pluripotent cells follows the basic principles of routine tissue culture, requiring a humidified, temperature-controlled environment with supplemental carbon dioxide. However, specific culture conditions are recommended to enhance the propagation of pluripotent cells. For example, FGF2 treatment in low oxygen conditions has been shown to increase the expression of pluripotency induction genes and may improve iPS cell generation.[31] To maintain pluripotency, ES/iPS cells must be kept isolated from differentiating cells in the colony to prevent cell signaling that can stimulate further differentiation. Conditions for propagation of pluripotent cells can vary widely by species, and have not yet been optimized for the horse, but the following specialized components have been used.

Leukemia inhibitory factor (LIF) is an interleukin class 6 cytokine that prevents ES/iPS cells from differentiating. LIF functions through activation of the JAK-STAT pathway. In the early embryo, LIF is produced by trophectoderm cells, while the LIF receptor is expressed by the inner cell mass of the blastocyst. Isolation of the inner cell mass removes ES cells from their endogenous source, necessitating supplementation of LIF through either recombinant protein or another LIF-expressing cell type. Media supplementation with recombinant LIF has been used in some, but not all, putative equine ES/iPS cell expansion culture systems to maintain cells in an undifferentiated state.

Feeder cells provide an alternate source of LIF for maintenance of pluripotent cells. Feeder cells can be derived from a variety of sources including mouse embryonic fibroblasts (MEF), equine embryonic fibroblasts (EEF), JK1 feeder cells, SNL76/7 cells, and STO cells. Feeder cells need to be irradiated or treated with mitomycin-c to inhibit their replication before use. Different types of feeder cells have been used for propagation of equine ES/iPS cells, but conditions are not yet optimized.

Bone morphogenetic proteins (BMP) are a family of growth factor proteins that contribute to propagation of pluripotent cells without differentiation and are very important in embryonic patterning and skeletal development. BMPs function through activation of the SMAD pathway. Serum supplies endogenous BMPs or media can be supplemented with recombinant BMP proteins if serum-free conditions are used. Serum is an important media component of all equine ES cell culture protocols to date.

CHARACTERIZATION OF ES/iPS CELLS AND EVALUATION OF PLURIPOTENCY
Cellular Morphology

Pluripotent cells have a unique appearance when grown in culture that can be used as an initial screen during colony selection. ES/iPS cells typically have a round shape, with large nucleolus and scant cytoplasm (**Fig. 1**). Colonies of human ES cells have sharp edges and are flat with tightly packed cells. In contrast, mouse colonies are less flat and tend to aggregate and become 3-dimensional. iPS colonies appear morphologically similar to the phenotype of ES cells from their respective species. Equine pluripotent cells are similar in morphologic appearance to human ES cells.[19] ES/iPS cells are mitotically active, leading to self-renewal and spontaneous differentiation, necessitating frequent passage to maintain the cells in a pluripotent state.

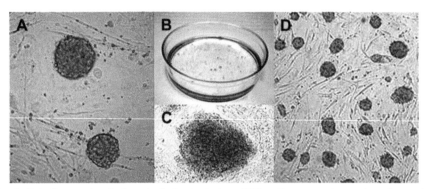

Fig. 1. Putative equine induced pluripotent stem (iPS) cells on a primary transformation plate (*A–C*) and after culture for 13 passages (*D*). The putative equine iPS colonies (*A, D*) are morphologically similar to human iPS cell colonies and are positive for alkaline phosphatase staining (*B, C*). (*Courtesy of* Lauren V. Schnabel, DVM, Ithaca, NY.)

Embryoid body (EB) formation is one assay that has been used as evidence of pluripotency in putative ES/iPS cells. Embryoid bodies are spherical cell aggregates that contain a variety of differentiated cell types on the outer surface with a core of mitotically active ES cells. EBs can be induced to form in culture by suspending ES/iPS cells within a hanging drop, by the use of nonadherent plasticware, or through use of spinner flasks that reduce normal ES cellular attachment. Although not definitive for ES/iPS validation, EB formation suggests that cells have the potential to form multiple tissues.

In vitro differentiation assays previously described for evaluating pluripotency in human and murine ES cells have been used in the validation of putative equine ES/iPS cells. Evidence of in vitro differentiation of equine-derived cells into all 3 primary germ layers has been reported.[4,7] However, without evidence of in vivo differentiation, the value of in vitro assays to demonstrate pluripotency is questionable.

Antibody reaction is one of the greatest challenges in characterizing putative ES/iPS cells. Reagents need to be developed that will accurately detect specific proteins required for validation of pluripotency in the species of interest. This is particularly true in the horse. Antibodies that are not specifically designed to identify the equine epitope need to be carefully validated for cross-species reactivity and specificity for the target equine protein. Since only about 4% of human antibodies react with their equivalent equine protein, most antihuman antibodies are not suitable for use in validation of cells derived from horses.[32] Further, cross-species variability in pluripotency markers makes definitive validation of putative equine ES/iPS cells using antibody profiling difficult.[8] Many of the nonequine antibodies that have been tried for equine ES/iPS cell immunohistochemical analysis include antibodies directed against Oct4, SSEA1, SSEA4, SSEA4, TRA-1-60, and TRA-1-81 proteins.[4] In this particular study, antibodies reacted not only with the equine inner cell mass, but also with equine trophoblast cells, suggesting these antibodies are not specific to proteins found exclusively on ES cells. Given this information, it is safe to conclude that currently available nonequine antibodies are not adequate to demonstrate pluripotency in equine cells.

Histologic assays that employ stains such as alkaline phosphatase are not specific for pluripotency. Most tissues in the body have alkaline phosphatase activity, and some tissues such as kidney, liver, and bone have increased levels of alkaline phosphatase. Previous studies have reported reactivity of antibodies directed against the specific alkaline phosphatase found in embryonic stem cells with many adult cell types, demonstrating the nonspecific nature of this assay.[33] Although alkaline phosphatase staining can provide supportive evidence that cells are in a pluripotent state, it is not specific or definitive.

Teratoma formation is a more stringent assay for assessment of cellular pluripotency. Teratomas are tumors containing cell types representative of all 3 primary germ layers. Unlike most tumors that contain only one cell type, teratomas can contain a variety of tissue types including cartilage, bone, skin, hair, and glandular tissue. The assay is typically performed by injection of putative ES/iPS cells into immunodeficient mice. In species other than mice, teratoma formation is the definitive test to validate that ES/iPS cell lines are pluripotent.

Recently, a report described generation of equine iPS cells derived from fetal fibroblasts that were able to form complex teratomas in NOD/SCID mice.[19] This group used many novel techniques including a nonviral, *piggyBac* transposon-based method to deliver transgenes containing the reprogramming factors Oct4, Sox2, Klf4 and c-Myc into horse cells. Reprogrammed equine iPS cells were under the influence of a tetracycline-inducible promoter and were identifiable by constitutive green fluorescent protein expression. Following transplantation into NOD/SCID mice, the researchers continued to feed recipient mice doxycycline for several weeks to prolong pluripotency gene expression in the iPS cell transplants, enhancing teratoma formation. The authors readily discuss the pitfalls of their study, but this report represents a major advance in the field of equine ES/iPS research.

Prior to this publication, there had been no reports of equine ES or iPS cells forming teratomas in immunocopromised mice. Some groups suggested that the horse was a species with a unique ability to avoid teratoma formation when ES cells are injected, making equine ES-like cells a potentially suitable source of cells for therapeutic use.[3,4,7] An alternate explanation was that a true equine ES/iPS cell line had not yet successfully been isolated. It was difficult to reconcile the argument that horse ES/iPS cell lines were unique when ES/iPS cells isolated from a number of mammalian species including cattle, swine, mice, and people all yielded teratomas under similar conditions.[8] It is now known that teratoma formation can occur in equine pluripotent cells.

Generation of offspring through chimera/tetraploid complementation assays is an even more rigorous test of pluripotency than teratoma formation. Murine studies have a distinct advantage here, with accurate methods of tracking cell fate in vivo. Through direct injection of putative ES/iPS cells into mouse trophoblasts, viable chimeric pups can be produced with 10% to 90% contribution to the chimeric pups' tissues. Germ-line transmission is possible in the chimera and can be tracked in subsequent generations using coat color analysis.

In mice, tetraploid complementation is the gold standard for validation of ES cell pluripotency. Tetraploid complementation is performed using blastocysts with twice the normal number of chromosomes (tetraploid). Putative ES/iPS cells are then injected into the tetraploid blastocysts, which then form whole, nonchimeric, fertile mice. The offspring are entirely derived from the injected ES/iPS cells. The tetraploid cells of the blastocysts contribute only to the formation of extraembryonic tissues such as the fetal portion of the placenta.

DNA/chromatin methylation patterns and the role of epigenetics have become important areas of research in studies related to cellular differentiation. In general, chromatin structure and organization have important effects on the expression of genes as cells pass through differentiation or reprogramming. Decreased cytosine methylation is often noted in the DNA promoter regions of genes that are transcriptionally active. Similarly, the H3 histones may also be demethylated when genes become active, opening the chromatin and making the DNA more accessible to transcriptional machinery. The addition of agents that alter chromatin structure and DNA methylation states have been used as media supplements to enhance the reprogramming of iPS cells.[34]

CLINICAL TRIALS

Much excitement has been generated about the transition of ES/iPS cell research into both human and equine clinical applications. The Geron Company (Menlo Park, CA, USA) has just received US Food and Drug Administration (FDA) approval for phase 1 safety trials in people using oligodendrocyte precursor cells (GRNOPC1), derived from human ES cells. Transplantation studies have begun in clinical patients. The original FDA approval was delayed when small numbers of microscopic cysts were found in the spinal cords of experimental rats treated with the human GRNOPC1cells. Initial safety studies will be conducted in paraplegic human patients with complete loss of sensory and neurologic function following subacute (<2 weeks) spinal cord injuries, before significant scar tissue has formed.

In horses, there is a published report of injection of undifferentiated equine ES-like cells into experimentally induced tendon lesions.[3] In that study, ES-like cells displayed longer survival and more extensive migration throughout areas of tendon damage than the adult bone marrow-derived cell treatment group. However, the study reported no significant histologic differences in tendon architecture between the serum control group and both cell (adult bone marrow and ES-like) therapy groups, suggesting the contribution of implanted cells to the repair was minimal at the time of histologic analysis.

Several companies are in the development process of commercializing equine ES/iPS therapies. The Celavet Company (Oxnard, CA, USA) has developed a line of putative ES-like cells that have been implanted in an equine experimental model of collagenase-induced superficial digital flexor tendonitis.[20] A multicenter, blinded, randomized controlled study using the Celavet cell lines in clinical cases of equine tendonitis is awaiting final FDA approval. ViaGen (Austin, TX, USA), Incorporated, along with researchers from the Monash Institute of Medical Research, is also developing commercial lines of reprogrammed equine cells (ViaGen.com) for clinical use.

Although little information is currently available on the translation of ES/iPS cells to the clinics, the rapid advances being made in basic research will likely lead to effective, regenerative cell-based products in the near future. The equine patient stands to gain tremendous benefit from ES/iPS applications, when safe, fully validated products become available for enhanced repair of musculoskeletal injuries. However, care needs to be exercised in preclinical analysis to ensure accurate classification of ES/iPS cell phenotype and subsequent differentiation into the desired cell product before implantation.

REFERENCES

1. Thomson JA, Itskovitz-Eldor J, Shapiro SS, et al. Embryonic stem cell lines derived from human blastocysts. Science 1998;282(5391):1145–7.
2. Kaufman MH, Robertson EJ, Handyside AH, et al. Establishment of pluripotential cell lines from haploid mouse embryos. J Embryol Exp Morphol 1983;73:249–61.
3. Guest DJ, Smith MR, Allen WR. Equine embryonic stem-like cells and mesenchymal stromal cells have different survival rates and migration patterns following their injection into damaged superficial digital flexor tendon. Equine Vet J 2010; 42(7):636–42.

4. Guest DJ, Allen WR. Expression of cell surface antigens and embryonic stem cell pluripotency genes in equine blastocysts. Stem Cells Dev 2007;16(5):789–96.
5. Saito S, Sawai K, Minamihashi A, et al. Derivation, maintenance, and induction of the differentiation in vitro of equine embryonic stem cells. Methods Mol Biol 2006; 329:59–79.
6. Saito S, Ugai H, Sawai K, et al. Isolation of embryonic stem-like cells from equine blastocysts and their differentiation in vitro. FEBS Lett 2002;531(3):389–96.
7. Li X, Zhou SG, Imreh MP, et al. Horse embryonic stem cell lines from the proliferation of inner cell mass cells. Stem Cells Dev 2006;15(4):523–31.
8. Paris DB, Stout TA. Equine embryos and embryonic stem cells: defining reliable markers of pluripotency. Theriogenology 2010;74(4):516–24.
9. Laurent LC, Ulitsky I, Slavin I, et al. Dynamic changes in the copy number of pluripotency and cell proliferation genes in human ESCs and iPSCs during reprogramming and time in culture. Cell Stem Cell 2011;8(1):106–18.
10. Ledermann B, Burki K. Establishment of a germ-line competent C57BL/6 embryonic stem cell line. Exp Cell Res 1991;197(2):254–8.
11. Kim JB, Zaehres H, Wu G, et al. Pluripotent stem cells induced from adult neural stem cells by reprogramming with two factors. Nature 2008;454(7204):646–50.
12. Kunisato A, Wakatsuki M, Kodama Y, et al. Generation of induced pluripotent stem cells by efficient reprogramming of adult bone marrow cells. Stem Cells Dev 2010;19(2):229–38.
13. Takahashi K, Yamanaka S. Induction of pluripotent stem cells from mouse embryonic and adult fibroblast cultures by defined factors. Cell 2006;126(4):663–76.
14. Yu J, Vodyanik MA, Smuga-Otto K, et al. Induced pluripotent stem cell lines derived from human somatic cells. Science 2007;318(5858):1917–20.
15. Takahashi K, Tanabe K, Ohnuki M, et al. Induction of pluripotent stem cells from adult human fibroblasts by defined factors. Cell 2007;131(5):861–72.
16. Stadtfeld M, Nagaya M, Utikal J, et al. Induced pluripotent stem cells generated without viral integration. Science 2008;322(5903):945–9.
17. Kim D, Kim CH, Moon JI, et al. Generation of human induced pluripotent stem cells by direct delivery of reprogramming proteins. Cell Stem Cell 2009;4(6):472–6.
18. Warren L, Manos PD, Ahfeldt T, et al. Highly efficient reprogramming to pluripotency and directed differentiation of human cells with synthetic modified mRNA. Cell Stem Cell 2010;7(5):618–30.
19. Nagy K, Sung HK, Zhang P, et al. Induced pluripotent stem cell lines derived from equine fibroblasts. Stem Cell Rev 2011. DOI: 10.1007/s12015-011-9239-5.
20. Watts AE, Yeager AE, Kopyov OV, et al. Fetal derived embryonic-like stem cells improve healing in a large animal flexor tendonitis model. Stem Cell Res Ther 2011;2(1):4.
21. Gutierrez-Aranda I, Ramos-Mejia V, Bueno C, et al. Human induced pluripotent stem cells develop teratoma more efficiently and faster than human embryonic stem cells regardless the site of injection. Stem Cells 2010;28(9):1568–70.
22. Niwa H, Miyazaki J, Smith AG. Quantitative expression of Oct-3/4 defines differentiation, dedifferentiation, or self-renewal of ES cells. Nat Genet 2000;24(4):372–6.
23. Kim JB, Sebastiano V, Wu G, et al. Oct4-induced pluripotency in adult neural stem cells. Cell 2009;136(3):411–9.
24. Episkopou V. SOX2 functions in adult neural stem cells. Trends Neurosci 2005; 28(5):219–21.
25. Masui S, Nakatake Y, Toyooka Y, et al. Pluripotency governed by Sox2 via regulation of Oct3/4 expression in mouse embryonic stem cells. Nat Cell Biol 2007; 9(6):625–35.

26. Mitsui K, Tokuzawa Y, Itoh H, et al. The homeoprotein Nanog is required for maintenance of pluripotency in mouse epiblast and ES cells. Cell 2003;113(5):631–42.
27. Wernig M, Meissner A, Foreman R, et al. In vitro reprogramming of fibroblasts into a pluripotent ES-cell-like state. Nature 2007;448(7151):318–24.
28. Darr H, Mayshar Y, Benvenisty N. Overexpression of NANOG in human ES cells enables feeder-free growth while inducing primitive ectoderm features. Development 2006;133(6):1193–201.
29. Lin T, Chao C, Saito S, et al. p53 induces differentiation of mouse embryonic stem cells by suppressing Nanog expression. Nat Cell Biol 2005;7(2):165–71.
30. Cotterman R, Jin VX, Krig SR, et al. N-Myc regulates a widespread euchromatic program in the human genome partially independent of its role as a classical transcription factor. Cancer Res 2008;68(23):9654–62.
31. Page RL, Ambady S, Holmes WF, et al. Induction of stem cell gene expression in adult human fibroblasts without transgenes. Cloning Stem Cells 2009;11(3): 417–26.
32. Ibrahim S, Saunders K, Kydd JH, et al. Screening of anti-human leukocyte monoclonal antibodies for reactivity with equine leukocytes. Vet Immunol Immunopathol 2007;119:63–80.
33. Hass PE, Wada HG, Herman MM, et al. Alkaline phosphatase of mouse teratoma stem cells: immunochemical and structural evidence for its identity as a somatic gene product. Proc Natl Acad Sci U S A 1979;76(3):1164–8.
34. Sumer H, Liu J, Verma PJ. The use of signalling pathway inhibitors and chromatin modifiers for enhancing pluripotency. Theriogenology 2010;74(4):525–33.

Mesenchymal Stem Cells: Characteristics, Sources, and Mechanisms of Action

Matthew C. Stewart, BVSc, MVetClinStud, PhD*,
Allison A. Stewart, DVM, MS

KEYWORDS

- Mesenchymal stem cell • Differentiation • Osteogenesis
- Chondrogenesis

Friedenstein and colleagues[1] originally described mesenchymal stem cells (MSC) almost 40 years ago. In bone marrow, MSCs are a component of the marrow stromal cell population that collectively supports hematopoietic stem cell persistence and differentiation. However, since this initial description, it is now recognized that MSCs reside in small numbers in many, if not all, adult tissues and organs and play an active role in the homeostasis of these sites. Given that MSCs can be reliable isolated and expanded from a wide range of adult tissue sources, are capable of differentiating into several musculoskeletal tissue types, and have notable immunomodulatory and antiinflammatory activities, these cells have been the subject of great interest in the biomedical research community since Friedenstein's discovery.

CHARACTERIZATION OF MSCs

The original criteria used to identify MSCs involved their ability to adhere to plastic substrates, the capacity for substantial clonal expansion, and the ability to differentiate along several mesenchymal cell lineages.[1,2]

Adherence to tissue culture plastic is a very nonspecific cellular property, but adhesion does exclude cell subpopulations within the marrow cavity that are committed to the hematopoietic lineages. Separation of nucleated cell populations by centrifugation over Percoll or Ficoll density gradients increases the stem cell concentration of initial preparations and is a standard component of many isolation protocols,[3–6] although gravity sedimentation has been advocated as a more effective method for progenitor

The authors have nothing to disclose.
Department of Veterinary Clinical Medicine, College of Veterinary Medicine, University of Illinois, 1008 West Hazelwood Drive, Urbana, IL 61802, USA
* Corresponding author.
E-mail address: matt1@illinois.edu

concentration.[7] The capacity for sustained proliferation is the basis for the routine isolation of MSCs by in vitro clonal expansion (**Fig. 1**); more differentiated cell types that might be included in biologic samples collected for MSC isolation are unable to contribute to the expanded cell population over several in vitro passages, resulting in a predominance of stem cells in the final preparation.

Although MSCs are capable of considerable cell division, this capacity is not unlimited. In this respect, MSCs differ from embryonic stem cells. In vivo, adult stem cells are in a near-quiescent state;[8] cell divisions are rare events. In vitro MSC expansion constitutes a marked and sustained increase in proliferation, resulting in replicative senescence. The rate and persistence of MSC proliferation appears to vary between tissue sources[9–11] and between different anatomic locations of the same tissue.[12] In general, bone marrow–derived progenitors have less proliferative capacity than MSCs derived from other tissues.[9,11,13] This difference may reflect differential in vivo proliferation of these MSC populations before collection and ex vivo expansion assays.

MSC replicative senescence is associated with a loss of multipotency[14,15] and impacts the critical ability of stem cells to home to sites of injury and inflammation.[16] This phenomenon is critical to applications that require extensive ex vivo MSC expansion before reimplantation. The onset and effects of replicative senescence can be mitigated by expanding MSCs in the presence of fibroblast growth factor 2 (FGF2).[17,18] FGF2 is now routinely added to MSC growth media.[19–21] Hypoxic culture conditions also accelerate MSC proliferation while maintaining a stem cell state,[22] whereas expansion in reduced glucose culture medium reduces MSC apoptosis and increases colony formation and size.[15]

Multi-Lineage Differentiation

The capacity for differentiation along several mesenchymal cell lineages is an integral component of the MSC phenotype. This characteristic is routinely assayed for in experimental studies and is the basis for tissue-engineering applications of MSCs for musculoskeletal repair and regeneration.

Generally, trilineage differentiation capacity is assessed because the in vitro requirements for osteogenic, chondrogenic, and adipogenic differentiation and appropriate phenotype-specific assays for these lineages are well characterized. In brief, osteogenic differentiation requires monolayer culture in serum-containing medium supplemented with β-glycerophosphate, dexamethasone and ascorbic acid. Osteogenic

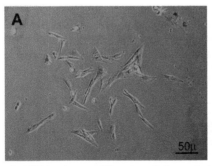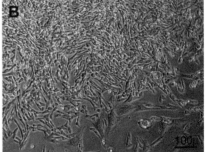

Fig. 1. MSC in vitro proliferation. Cells seeded at low density adhere to tissue culture plastic within 3 to 4 days and are initially evident as sparse clusters of small numbers of cells (*A*). After several days, rapid MSC proliferation results in large colony formation. The edge of a large, established colony is shown in (*B*).

differentiation occurs as cells reach confluence and aggregate to form 3-dimensional nodules. Bone morphogenetic proteins (BMP) can be added to the osteogenic medium to accelerate osteogenic differentiation and increase matrix mineralization. The osteogenic phenotype is identified by assaying for the deposition of mineralized matrix (von Kossa staining, alizarin red staining; **Fig. 2**A), increased alkaline phosphatase (ALP) activity, and upregulation of osteoblast-specific genes, such as Runx2, Osterix, osteopontin, osteonectin, bone sialic protein, and ALP.

Chondrogenic differentiation requires a 3-dimensional culture system; pellet or micromass cultures are used most commonly. MSC pellets are cultured in serum-free medium supplemented with ascorbic acid and insulin, transferrin, and selenium and treated with a transforming growth factor-β or BMPs. The chondrogenic phenotype is assayed by the secretion and deposition of the collagen type II protein (enzyme-linked immunosorbent assay); sulfated glycosaminoglycans (dimethylmethylene blue binding) or aggrecan (Western blotting); matrix staining for sulfated glycosaminoglycans (alcian blue, toluidine blue, or safranin O; see **Fig. 2**B) and collagen type II immunohistochemistry; and by transcriptional profiling for chondrocyte-specific genes, such

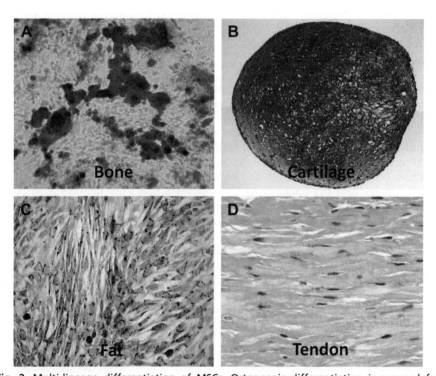

Fig. 2. Multi-lineage differentiation of MSCs. Osteogenic differentiation is assessed for staining for mineralized matrix in the cell layer by alizarin red (*A*). Chondrogenic differentiation is assayed using a pellet culture model. Sulfated glycosaminoglycans within the cartilaginous extracellular matrix are stained with toluidine blue (*B*). Adipogenic differentiation is determined by staining intracellular lipid-filled vacuoles with oil red O (*C*). Assays for tenogenic differentiation is less well defined; however, cellular and matrix alignment, as in the native tissue, can be histologically assessed, as seen in this bioreactor-generated bone marrow MSC construct (*D*). (*Courtesy of* Roger Smith, Department of Veterinary Clinical Sciences, The Royal Veterinary College, University of London, UK [*A, D*].)

as Sox 9, collagen type II, aggrecan, and link protein mRNAs. Induction of the hypertrophic chondrocytic phenotype is generally monitored by assaying ALP activity and upregulation of collagen type X and ALP mRNAs.

For adipogenic differentiation, cells are incubated as monolayers in medium and 10% serum, supplemented with dexamethasone, isobutylmethylxanthine (IBMX), and insulin. In some protocols, indomethacin is also included in adipogenic medium. IBMX sensitizes the cells to insulin, whereas insulin itself stimulates lipid synthesis and accumulation within intracellular vacuoles. Adipogenic differentiation is assessed by staining the lipid-filled vacuoles with oil-red-O (see **Fig. 2**C) and by the upregulation of the adipocyte-specific transcription factor, PPARγ.

Assessing MSC differentiation along the tenogenic lineage is less established, largely because phenotype-specific markers are not well defined. However, recent studies have induced tenogenic differentiation in serum-supplemented medium with growth and differentiation factor 5 (GDF-5) or GDF-7/BMP-12.[23,24] Induction of the tenocytic phenotype can be assayed by assessing cellular orientation (see **Fig. 2**D); measuring collagen secretion (hydroxyl-proline measurement); and transcriptional upregulation of scleraxis (a tenocyte-specific transcription factor), tenomodulin, tenascin-C, Smad-8 and extracellular matrix genes, collagen types I and II, aggrecan, and decorin.[24–26] Protocols have also been developed to stimulate MSC differentiation along neurogenic, myogenic, and endothelial pathways,[27] but these topics are beyond the subject matter of this review.

Cell Surface Marker Profiling

In addition to adhesion, proliferation, and multi-lineage differentiation, attempts have been made to formalize MSC identification on the basis of cell surface markers as analyzed by fluorescence-activated cell sorting or flow cytometry. The obvious appeal of this immunophenotyping approach lies in the fact that nominally purified populations of surface marker–characterized MSCs could be rapidly isolated from mixed-cell primary preparations (aspirates, tissue digests, and body fluids) and isolation protocols could be standardized. The emphasis for MSC immunophenotyping has been on developing the capacity to discriminate MSCs from non-MSCs in bone marrow aspirates. A panel of negative markers has been developed to identify and exclude non-MSC marrow populations, such as hematopoietic stem cells (cluster of differentiation [CD] 34 and CD117), erythroid precursors (glycophorin-A), immune/myeloid cells (CD11b), the B cell lineage (CD19 and CD45), endothelial cells (CD31), monocytes (CD14), and lymphocytes major histocompatibility complex II.[28,29]

Identifying one or more surface markers that will positively identify MSCs has proven to be more challenging, partly because there are clear interspecies differences in cell surface marker expression and because the immunophenotype of putative MSCs changes with time in culture.[5,30,31] A recent review of the literature suggested that three markers be used for human MSC purification: Stro1, CD73, and CD106.[29] Stro1 reliably identifies colony-forming precursor cells from marrow.[32] Two monoclonal antibodies have been developed to target CD73, or lymphocyte-vascular adhesion protein 2, with specificity for mesenchymal tissue–derived cells.[33] These antibodies do not recognize osteoblasts or hematopoietic stem cells, which is particularly useful for processing bone marrow aspirates. VCAM-1, or CD106, is expressed by endothelial and perivascular cells.[30] CD106 expression by MSCs probably reflects their localization near vessels and relates to their ability to mobilize into the vasculature with appropriate chemotactic cues.

The situation in horses and other nonhuman species is much less clear. Work in this field has been restricted by a lack of validated antibodies to recognize nonhuman/rodent surface markers, as well as biologic differences between species. As an example, the epitope recognized by the Stro1 antibody appears to be human specific, and its value in other species is unclear. A recent review of equine MSC immunophenotyping recommended that equine MSCs should express CD29, CD44, and CD90.[28] CD29 is a β integrin, CD44 is a hyaluronate receptor; both are highly expressed by equine bone marrow–derived MSCs in vitro,[5] but both are widely expressed across connective tissue cell types. In the analysis by Kolf and colleagues,[29] none of the epitopes recommended for equine MSC identification made the cut for human stem cell analyses because of insufficient specificity for MSCs. Further, there is a large body of evidence demonstrating that immunophenotypically similar MSC populations from different tissue sources have very divergent capacities for differentiation along osteogenic, chondrogenic, and adipogenic lineages.[10,34–38] Clearly, a considerable amount of work still needs to be done to develop a reliable protocol for equine MSC immunophenotyping and isolation, as well as determining whether any given immunophenotype is clinically superior to unsorted or alternatively sorted cell populations.

SOURCES OF MSCs

Much of the early work on MSC biology was focused on bone marrow–derived cells, but there is an increasing appreciation that MSCs are present in variably low numbers in many tissues and body fluids. As more is learned about these alternative MSC sources, opportunities for less complex specimen collection and source-specific clinical applications have been developed.

The Niche Concept

Accepting that MSCs reside in many, if not all, tissues and organs, a complex and highly regulated system is necessary to ensure that stem cells are maintained in an undifferentiated state, proliferate at a rate appropriate for the needs of downstream progenitor cells, and support intrinsic self-renewal. These regulatory systems are spatially organized into what are termed stem cell niches. Niches provide the collective physical, cell contact-mediated, and secretory factor stimuli to maintain stem cell populations, control stem cell proliferative activity and the appropriate generation of daughter cell progenitors and new stem cells (asymmetric division). As examples, the hematopoietic stem cell (HSC) niche is located on the endosteal surfaces of trabecular bone, in contact with endosteal osteoblasts and endothelial cells lining marrow cavity vessels[39]; epithelial stem cells are located specifically at the follicular bulge of the hair follicle root sheath[40]; the intestinal stem cell niche is located at the base of intestinal crypts adjacent to Paneth cells that are active in innate immune responses at the intestinal surface[41]; and skeletal muscle stem cells reside immediately adjacent to the myofiber plasma membranes, within the muscle satellite cell population.[42]

In addition to the stem cell population itself, niches contain one or more distinct support cell populations that provide the soluble and cell contact-mediated signals required to maintain stem cell functions. Generally speaking, stem cell niches are located close to vasculature, presumably to ensure adequate nutrition and facilitate progenitor cell migration through the vascular system, and are in highly protected sites relative to the positions of their more differentiated offspring. In contrast to the niche descriptions previously mentioned, the specific locations and features of the MSC niche are not currently known, apart from the strong likelihood that they are within the perivascular microenvironment.[29] Given that MSC-like populations have been successfully isolated from many tissues and organs of nonmesodermal origin,[43] the MSC niches must be highly adaptable to a variety of cellular and matrix contexts.

From a clinical perspective, stem cell niches are critical for maintaining effective stem cell reserves. Loss or dysregulation of niche activity has been linked to ageing, degenerative diseases, and tumor development.[44] Further, specimen collection for stem cell isolation must access niche sites to be successful.

Bone Marrow MSCs

As previously mentioned, bone marrow MSCs (BM MSC) are a subpopulation of the stromal cells that line the endosteal surface of the marrow space and form the hematopoietic stem cell niche. Using human specimens, Sachetti and colleagues[45] specifically identified bone marrow osteoprogenitor cells as being restricted to a melanoma-associated cell adhesion molecule/CD146-positive population located within the subendothelial layer of sinusoidal walls, immediately adjacent the HSC niche. Cells in many respects identical to BM MSCs can be isolated from trabecular and compact bone[46–48] and from nonhematopoietic bone marrow sites, such as the femoral head,[49] strongly suggesting that BM BSC populations exist in close association with trabecular bone surfaces, distinct from HSC niche sites.

In horses, BM MSCs are routinely isolated from marrow aspirates collected from the tuber coxae[13,50] or sternebrae.[6,51] A recent study determined that the fifth sternebra was the most reliable and safest site for aspiration.[52] Although, intuitively, more is better, this study also determined that the first 5 mL of an aspirate is most enriched for MSCs. In practice, single aspirate volumes of 10 to 20 mL are probably adequate. The methods for equine BM MSC collection and culture are covered in detail in the article by Taylor and Clegg elsewhere in this issue.

Equine BM MSCs have been used experimentally to repair collagenase-induced tendon lesions[53] and surgically created articular cartilage defects[54,55] with limited success; however, the results following BM MSC administration in clinical cases of flexor tendon strain injuries[56–58] and arthritis involving injury to intraarticular soft-tissue structures[59] are more impressive. These topics are covered in more detail by Alves and colleagues and by Frisbie and Stewart elsewhere in this issue.

Adipose Tissue MSCs

MSCs derived from adipose tissue (AD MSC) have become a highly attractive alternative to BM MSCs in recent years, largely due to the ease of tissue collection, high initial cell yields and robust in vitro proliferative capacity.[9,11,13,60] Although the specific details have not been determined, the AD MSC niche is likely to be perivascular, as in other tissues, because stem cell yields from equine adipose tissue have been correlated with vascular density.[61] Detailed coverage of adipose tissue collection and AD MSC isolation is provided by Taylor and Clegg elsewhere in this issue.

AD MSCs are capable of multi-lineage differentiation, both in vitro and in vivo,[62,63] but the weight of evidence from several species,[34,36,38,64–66] including the horse,[11,67–69] indicates that AD MSCs are biosynthetically less capable of generating osseous or cartilaginous tissues than are BM MSC and other MSC populations. This finding might be associated with an altered responsiveness of AD MSCs to transforming growth factor (TGF) β and BMP ligand stimulation because BMP-6 supplementation significantly increases chondrogenic differentiation by these cells.[62,70] In contrast, AD MSCs appear to be particularly potent as immunomodulatory agents, as assessed in immune-mediated arthritis models,[71] and in vitro lymphocyte activation assays.[72] Accepting the expediency of adipose tissue collection, AD MSCs might be specifically indicated for antiinflammatory and immunosuppressive applications rather than tissue regeneration purposes. Further, there is evidence that the regenerative capacities of AD MSCs vary with location.[12] Accepting that the tail butt area is an expedient site for collection, other adipose tissue locations might contain AD MSCs with more desirable biologic properties for specific clinical applications. As an example, AD MSCs from the infrapatellar fat pad appear to be specifically preprogrammed for chondrogenic differentiation.[12,73]

Umbilical Cord Blood and Wharton Jelly MSCs

Collection of stem cells from umbilical cord blood (UCB) or from the collagen-rich matrix surrounding the umbilical vasculature, Wharton jelly,[74,75] is particularly attractive for clinical applications in performance horses. The collection procedure is entirely noninvasive, straightforward, and, self-evidently, the cells are obtained from a very young tissue source. Given the emphasis on pedigree records and the fact that valuable broodmares are usually monitored closely at the time of parturition, umbilical cord collection and donor-linked storage of UCB MSCs are feasible procedures. This strategy does require a secure cell bank to store the MSCs for anticipated future use. Several of these facilities have been opened in recent years.

The efficiency of MSC isolation and colony formation from UCB appears to be lower than that of BM and fat, but UCB MSCs exhibit higher and more sustained proliferation rates than other MSC sources.[9,37,75] This fact is likely a reflection of the neonatal age of the tissue source. The multi-lineage capacity of UCB MSCs is reported to be more restricted than BM or AD MSCs in that UCB cells are poor at undergoing adipogenic differentiation,[9,37,76] although this is not likely to be clinically important.

Tendon-Derived MSCs

Bi and colleagues[77] demonstrated the existence of MSCs in both murine and human tendon in 2007. The tendon-derived MSC (TD MSC) niche is located within the interfibrillar spaces. Transgenic studies in mice suggested that niche function is influenced by several small extracellular matrix proteins. TD MSCs are routinely isolated by first removing the paratenon, mincing or dicing the tendon matrix into small pieces, and digesting the tissue with collagenase. TD-MSCs are isolated from the resulting cell suspension by differential adherence and proliferation rates in monolayer culture.[78,79] TD MSCs have multi-lineage potential,[77,79] show particular affinity for acellular tendon matrix,[78] and, in in vivo differentiation assays, spontaneously regenerate tendonlike tissue structures.[77,80] In these respects, it is possible that TD MSCs are particularly suitable for the repair or regeneration of damaged tendon tissue.

Studies with equine cells indicate that TD MSCs colonize tendon matrix explants with greater efficiency than BM MSCs and synthesize greater quantities of ECM proteins after colonization.[78] The in vivo efficacy of TD MSC administration is currently being investigated in the equine collagenase-induced superficial digital flexor tendon (SDFT) model. Preliminary assessments indicate that intralesional TD MSC administration improves the organization of the repair tissue. Additional biochemical and biomechanical assessments are currently underway. This topic is covered in greater detail in the article by Alves and colleagues elsewhere in this issue.

Synovial MSCs

MSCs can be isolated from synovial membrane (SM) or from synovial fluid itself, although the initial cell yields from synovial fluid samples are extremely low. SM MSCs have been isolated and analyzed from rats,[81] rabbits,[82] pigs,[83] and cattle[84]; many studies have been performed using human samples because of the easy access to this tissue from total joint replacement surgeries.[10,35,85–88] SM MSCs presumably reside within the few cell layers of the synovial membrane itself. MSCs within synovial fluid could represent progenitor cells shed from membrane cells entering the joint space from the systemic circulation or could conceivably be derived from the population of stem cells residing within the articular cartilage.[89,90] Synovial MSCs are capable of considerable proliferative expansion and have multi-lineage differentiation potential; however, interest in this MSC source is based on the repeated observation that SM MSCs are more potently chondrogenic than MSCs from bone marrow, fat, or other common stem cell sources,[10,12,66,81] suggesting that this MSC source is particularly relevant for cartilage regeneration/repair. An in vivo rabbit cartilage defect study demonstrated effective cartilage regeneration following SM MSC implantation.[91]

The authors' own studies with equine cells have demonstrated that clinically useful chondroprogenitor cells can be grown from synovial fluid aspirates and from synovial membrane of horses. These cells exhibit rapid and persistent proliferation. Expanded cells are capable of chondrogenic differentiation in pellet cultures and are responsive to both BMP-2 and TGF-β1. Most importantly, chondrogenic SM MSCs do not express markers of the hypertrophic chondrocytic phenotype (ALP and collagen type X; personal observation, 2010),[92] suggesting that the specific phenotype of these cells is more consistent with a permanent, articular cartilage than to endochondral cartilage that is associated with bone formation.

Circulating MSCs

Several studies have identified low concentrations of multipotent MSCs in the blood samples of laboratory mammals[93,94] and, rarely, from humans.[93–95] Fibroblastic progenitor cells can be isolated from 30% to 60% of horses.[96,97] It is not known whether these circulating stem cells are derived from cells mobilized from bone marrow or other sites, or represent a small population of dedicated intravascular MSCs.

The concept that stem cells could be extracted directly from equine blood and concentrated for immediate clinical use is an attractive possibility. However, Ahern and colleagues[98] assessed the utility of apheresis to concentrate MSCs within the mononuclear cell fraction of peripheral blood and found that the apheresis process effectively removed or inactivated the MSCs. Until an efficient technique to separate and concentrate circulating MSCs from whole blood is developed, clinical applications for these cells will be unlikely.

MSC Concentrates

Isolating MSC populations from body fluids or tissue digests requires prolonged in vitro monolayer culture. In efforts to avoid this delay and to develop point-of-service therapies, concentrates of bone marrow aspirate (BMAC) and adipose-derived stromal vascular fractions (ADSVF) have been developed for clinical use. These preparations have the obvious advantage of being available for administration shortly after collection,[99] following centrifugation or tissue digestion, but the resultant cellular elements will contain a small minority of bona fide stem cells. BMAC is generated by processing bone marrow aspirate similarly to the technique used for platelet-rich plasma, with similar increases in cellular and growth factor concentrations.[100]

In people, BMAC has been used to augment bone defect infill,[101,102] nonunions,[103] cervical vertebral fusion,[104] and to treat osteonecrosis of the femoral head.[105] Based on these reports, there is a clear application for BMAC in the treatment of equine fracture repair. BMAC was also shown to improve articular cartilage defect repair following microfracture,[106] increasing the extent of defect infill, integration of repair tissue, and phenotypic characteristics of the tissue. BMAC implanted in a fibrin gel was also effective at repairing experimental cartilage defects in a rabbit model,[107] with impressive restoration of cellular organization, matrix collagen, and proteoglycan contents after 12 weeks. Bone marrow aspirate has also been used successfully in the equine collagenase-induced SDFT tendinitis model, with improved healing equivalent to that of BM MSC administration.[108]

ADVSF also has clinically useful benefits. In a study using human tissue specimens, the in vitro osteogenic capacities of ADVSF and culture-expanded AD MSCs were shown to be similar.[109] The clinical utility of ADSVF was assessed in the equine SDFT collagenase model by Nixon and colleagues[110] in 2007. Although there were no differences in tendon repair evident on ultrasonographic evaluations, ADSVF significantly improved tendon fiber orientation and reduced signs of inflammation at the injection sites. Although there were no obvious benefits from intraarticular ADSVF administration in the Colorado State University's carpal joint osteochondral fragment osteoarthritis model,[55] a large number of clinical case reports suggest that ADVSF is valuable for the treatment of equine tendinitis suspensory desmitis and osteoarthritis (www.vetstem.com/equine).[111]

MECHANISMS OF MSC ACTION: HOW DO MSCs WORK?
Primary Tissue Regeneration

Initial approaches to the use of MSCs for the treatment of musculoskeletal injuries were predicated on their ability to differentiate into the appropriate tissue types (see **Fig. 2**) and so directly stimulate regeneration of the damaged tissues.[112] Essentially, the expectation was that implanted or injected MSCs would colonize an injury site, differentiate into the appropriate mesenchymal tissue types, and affect repair. This expectation, in retrospect, was somewhat naïve for several reasons. Firstly, the processes of in vitro differentiation along osteogenic, chondrogenic, and other lineages recapitulate some of the qualitative aspects of tissue formation; however, the tissue-level complexities of mineralized bone or articular cartilage, as examples, are far from replicated in the in vitro assays routinely used to assess MSC differentiation. Using chondrogenesis as an informative example, although MSCs express the cardinal markers of the chondrocytic phenotype in vitro, their transcriptional profiles of chondrogenic MSCs and of intrinsic stem cell–mediated cartilage repair tissue in vivo are markedly different from that of fully differentiated articular chondrocytes.[113,114] Further, although the levels of chondrocyte-specific mRNA transcript expression (for example, collagen type II and aggrecan) by MSCs often match or exceed those of articular chondrocytes, the biosynthesis and deposition of these matrix proteins by MSCs are generally far less than activities of differentiated chondrocytes. In the authors' own laboratory, MSC matrix synthesis is usually 30% to 50% of that secreted by analogous chondrocyte cultures, despite impressive transcriptional activity.[92]

Although in vitro differentiation potential is considered to be a central characteristic of MSCs, their in vitro capacity does not necessarily reflect the ability of these cells to differentiate in vivo as have been demonstrated for both synovial and adipose-derived stem cells.[36,115] To confuse matters further, qualitative indices of in vitro differentiation are not the sole domain of stem cell populations. Articular chondrocytes have considerable latent phenotypic plasticity in vitro,[116] and these fully differentiated cell types can also be induced to undergo convincing osteogenic differentiation with appropriate stimulation (**Fig. 3**). Clearly, evidence of in vitro differentiation is no guarantee of clinically useful in vivo performance. Cell-labeling studies suggest that MSCs implanted at sites of cartilage or tendon injury do not remain at the injury site. Quintavella and colleagues[117] documented extensive release of implanted MSCs from a cartilage

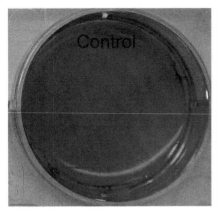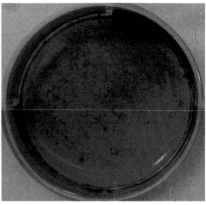

Fig. 3. In vitro transdifferentiation. Primary articular chondrocytes, a fully differentiated cell type, when grown as monolayers and maintained in osteogenic medium for 14 days, stain positively for mineralized matrix with alizarin red, as evident from the variably dark red staining of the cell layer in the treated (osteo) well, in contrast to the negative staining in the control well.

defect seven to 14 days after implantation, and cell-tracking studies in the equine SDFT collagenase model have shown that injected MSCs are lost from the injection site within four to six weeks (Allison Stewart, unpublished data, 2010).[118] In the study by Murphy and colleagues[119] that documented impressive meniscal regeneration in a caprine joint destabilization model, labeled MSCs were evident within the surface layers of the regenerated meniscal tissues, but the bulk of the repair tissue was populated by host cells. Finally, the considerable therapeutic benefits documented from the administration of BMAC and ADSVF (see previous discussion) suggest that highly concentrated MSC preparations are not required to stimulate tissue repair.

It should be pointed out that the direct involvement of MSCs in tissue repair differs in other contexts. As examples, in rat spinal cord injury models, implanted MSCs differentiate into various neuronal cell types and participate directly in cord regeneration/repair, with reduced astrocytic scar formation and improved functional outcomes,[120,121] and, in cardiac muscle repair following infarction, MSCs differentiate into endothelial cells to stimulate revascularization, undergo cardiomyogenic differentiation, and can also fuse with existing muscle cells to prolong the survival of the intrinsic cell population.[122]

MSC Effects on Other Cells

Accepting that MSCs are unlikely to be directly responsible for musculoskeletal tissue repair/regeneration, the critical importance of MSC paracrine activities is now being recognized. Much of this research is focused on the protection, repair, and regeneration of myocardium and the central nervous system (CNS) following ischemic insult, but mechanisms of action in these systems are likely relevant to MSC applications for musculoskeletal injuries.[123]

Comprehensive analyses of MSC secretory protein profiles[124] and transcriptosomes[125] indicate that MSCs secrete a diverse array of cytokines, growth factors, chemokines, and immunomodulatory proteins. In models of myocardial infarction and ischemia, MSCs improve myocardial repair through several mechanisms. Firstly, MSCs stimulate neovascularization of the infarct. Although there is some evidence for direct MSC differentiation or incorporation into the neovascular beds,[126,127] the majority of new endothelial cells are host derived and are stimulated by MSC secretion of the chemokine, SDF-1, and the angiogenic factor, VEGF.[128] In addition to stimulating revascularization, MSCs suppress fibrosis of the infarct, resulting in more compliant and functional ventricular muscle.[129,130] Exogenous MSCs also protect viable cardiomyocytes from postischemic apoptotic death and activate the intrinsic cardiac stem cell population to regenerate the damaged myocardium.[122] The paracrine nature of these effects has been demonstrated by conditioned medium experiments.[131,132]

The effects of MSC therapy on CNS lesions are very similar. Following cerebral ischemic insults, neural MSCs from the subventricular niche migrate to the ischemic lesion and protect resident neurons by stimulating neoangiogenesis through VEGF secretion and reducing apoptotic cell death at the ischemic lesion.[133,134] Locally delivered MSCs to spinal cord lesions exert similar neuron-sparing effects, with significant reductions in white matter loss and neuronal death and consequent improvements in clinical recovery.[135] This neuron-sparing activity is a consequence of soluble mediator release, since AD MSC-conditioned medium was also able to protect cerebellar neurons against apoptotic stimuli, through secreted IGF-1.[136]

Trophic factors can also work remotely. Pulmonary MSC emboli that develop following intravenous MSC administration protect infarcted myocardial cells by secreting an antiinflammatory factor, TSG-6.[137] Intramuscularly administered MSCs can also stimulate infracted myocardial revascularization by stimulating VEGF secretion by skeletal myocytes at the site of injection.[132]

The identification of MSC paracrine effects on immune cells has led to several stem cell–based clinical applications targeting immune-mediated and autoimmune conditions. Of particular interest, exposure to inflammatory cytokines, such as TNFα, IFN-γ, and IL-1β, stimulate MSC immunosuppressive activities,[137,138] suggesting a cellular negative feedback loop mediated by MSC responses that serves to dampen inflammatory reactions. Activated MSCs recruit T lymphocytes by chemokine secretion and reduce T lymphocyte proliferation, activation-antigen expression, and inflammatory cytokine secretion.[139,140] The immunomodulatory activities of MSCs are covered in greater detail in the article by Peroni and Borjesson elsewhere in this issue.

In summary, there is a wealth of evidence that MSCs secrete factors that promote angiogenesis, protect compromised host cells from apoptosis, and recruit and stimulate resident stem cells, while concurrently inhibiting inflammation and subsequent fibrosis. Although the collective effect of these activities might not result in authentic regeneration of musculoskeletal tissues, there is considerable promise that MSC therapies will substantially improve the functional quality of tissue repair, as has already been demonstrated in several studies addressing the treatment of equine flexor tendonitis, articular cartilage damage, and intraarticular soft-tissue injuries with these cells.

REFERENCES

1. Friedenstein AJ, Petrakova KV, Kurolesova AI, et al. Heterotopic of bone marrow. Analysis of precursor cells for osteogenic and hematopoietic tissues. Transplantation 1968;6:230–47.

2. Pittenger MF, Mackay AM, Beck SC, et al. Multilineage potential of adult human mesenchymal stem cells. Science 1999;284:143–7.

3. Yoo JU, Barthel TS, Mishimura K, et al. The chondrogenic potential of human bone-marrow-derived mesenchymal progenitor cells. J Bone Joint Surg Am 1998;80:1745–57.

4. Murphy JM, Dixon K, Beck S, et al. Reduced chondrogenic and adipogenic activity of mesenchymal stem cells from patients with advanced osteoarthritis. Arthritis Rheum 2002;46:704–13.

5. Radcliffe CH, Flaminio MJ, Fortier LA. Temporal analysis of equine bone marrow aspirate during establishment of putative mesenchymal progenitor cell populations. Stem Cells Dev 2009;19:269–82.

6. Bourzac C, Smith LC, Vincent P, et al. Isolation of equine bone marrow-derived mesenchymal stem cells: a comparison between three protocols. Equine Vet J 2010;42:519–27.

7. Carrancio S, Lopez-Holgado N, Sanchez-Guijo FM, et al. Optimization of mesenchymal stem cell expansion procedures by cell separation and culture conditions modification. Exp Hematol 2008;36:1014–21.

8. Orford KW, Scadden DT. Deconstructing stem cell self-renewal: genetic insights into cell-cycle regulation. Nat Rev Genet 2008;9:115–28.

9. Kern S, Eichler H, Stoeve J, et al. Comparative analysis of mesenchymal stem cells from bone marrow, umbilical cord blood, or adipose tissue. Stem Cells 2006;24:1294–301.

10. Shirasawa S, Sekiya I, Sakaguchi Y, et al. In vitro chondrogenesis of human synovium-derived mesenchymal stem cells: optimal condition and comparison with bone marrow-derived cells. J Cell Biochem 2006;97:84–97.

11. Vidal MA, Kilroy GE, Lopez MJ, et al. Characterization of equine adipose tissue-derived stromal cells: adipogenic and osteogenic capacity and comparison with bone marrow-derived mesenchymal stromal cells. Vet Surg 2007;36:613–22.

12. Mochizuki T, Muneta T, Sakaguchi Y, et al. Higher chondrogenic potential of fibrous synovium– and adipose synovium–derived cells compared with subcutaneous fat–derived cells. Arthritis Rheum 2006;54:843–53.

13. Colleoni S, Bottani E, Tessaro I, et al. Isolation, growth and differentiation of equine mesenchymal stem cells: effect of donor, source, amount of tissue and supplementation with basic fibroblast growth factor. Vet Res Commun 2009; 33:811–21.

14. Javazon EH, Beggs KJ, Flake AW. Mesenchymal stem cells: paradoxes of passaging. Exp Hematol 2004;32:414–25.

15. Stolzing A, Coleman N, Scutt A. Glucose-induced replicative senescence in mesenchymal stem cells. Rejuvenation Res 2006;9:31–5.

16. Rombouts WJ, Ploemacher RE. Primary murine MSC show highly efficient homing to the bone marrow but lose homing ability following culture. Leukemia 2003;17:160–70.

17. Tsutsumi S, Shimazu A, Miyazaki K, et al. Retention of multilineage differentiation potential of mesenchymal cells during proliferation in response to FGF. Biochem Biophys Res Commun 2001;288:413–9.

18. Zaragosi L, Ailhaud G, Dani C. Autocrine fibroblast growth factor 2 signaling is critical for self-renewal of human multipotent adipose-derived stem cells. Stem Cells 2006;24:2412–9.

19. Bianchi G, Banfi A, Mastrogiacomo M, et al. Ex vivo enrichment of mesenchymal cell progenitors by fibroblast growth factor 2. Exp Cell Res 2003;287:98–105.

20. Solchaga LA, Penick K, Porter JD, et al. FGF-2 enhances the mitotic and chondrogenic potentials of human adult bone marrow-derived mesenchymal stem cells. J Cell Physiol 2005;203:398–409.

21. Stewart AA, Byron CR, Pondenis H, et al. Effect of fibroblast growth factor-2 on equine mesenchymal stem cell monolayer expansion and chondrogenesis. Am J Vet Res 2007;68:941–5.

22. Grayson WL, Zhao F, Bunnell B, et al. Hypoxia enhances proliferation and tissue formation of human mesenchymal stem cells. Biochem Biophys Res Commun 2007;358:948–53.

23. Violini S, Ramelli P, Pisani LF, et al. Horse bone marrow mesenchymal stem cells express embryo stem cell markers and show the ability for tenogenic differentiation by in vitro exposure to BMP-12. BMC Cell Biol 2009;10:29.

24. Park A, Hogan MV, Kesturu GS, et al. Adipose-derived mesenchymal stem cells treated with growth differentiation factor-5 express tendon-specific markers. Tissue Eng Part A 2010;16:2941–51.

25. Halász K, Kassner A, Mörgelin M, et al. COMP acts as a catalyst in collagen fibrillogenesis. J Biol Chem 2007;26:31168–73.

26. Taylor SE, Vaughan-Thomas A, Clements DN, et al. Gene expression markers of tendon fibroblasts in normal and diseased tissue compared to monolayer and three dimensional culture systems. BMC Musculoskelet Disord 2009;10:27.

27. Barry FP, Murphy JM. Mesenchymal stem cells: clinical applications and biological characterization. Int J Biochem Cell Biol 2004;36:568–84.

28. De Schauwer C, Meyer E, Van de Walle GR, et al. Markers of stemness in equine mesenchymal stem cells: a plea for uniformity. Theriogenology 2010; 75:1431–43.

29. Kolf CM, Cho E, Tuan RS. Biology of adult mesenchymal stem cells: regulation of niche, self-renewal and differentiation. Arthritis Res Ther 2007;9:204.

30. Gronthos S, Zannettino AC, Hay SJ, et al. Molecular and cellular characterisation of highly purified stromal stem cells derived from human bone marrow. J Cell Sci 2003;116:1827–35.

31. Hackett CH, Flaminio MJ, Fortier LA. Analysis of CD14 expression levels in putative mesenchymal progenitor cells isolated from equine bone marrow. Stem Cells Dev 2011;20:721–35.

32. Simmons PJ, Torok-Storb B. Identification of stromal cell precursors in human bone marrow by a novel monoclonal antibody, STRO-1. Blood 1991;78:55–62.

33. Haynesworth SE, Baber MA, Caplan AI. Cell surface antigens on human marrow-derived mesenchymal cells are detected by monoclonal antibodies. Bone 1992;13:69–80.

34. Im G, Shin Y, Lee K. Do adipose tissue-derived mesenchymal stem cells have the same osteogenic and chondrogenic potential as bone marrow-derived cells? Osteoarthritis Cartilage 2005;13:845–53.

35. Djouad F, Bony C, Häupl T, et al. Transcriptional profiles discriminate bone marrow-derived and synovium-derived mesenchymal stem cells. Arthritis Res Ther 2005;7:R1304–15.

36. Park J, Gelse K, Frank S, et al. Transgene-activated mesenchymal cells for articular cartilage repair: a comparison of primary bone marrow-, perichondrium/periosteum- and fat-derived cells. J Gene Med 2006;8:112–25.

37. Rebelatto CK, Aguiar AM, Moretao MP, et al. Dissimilar differentiation of mesenchymal stem cells from bone marrow, umbilical cord blood, and adipose tissue. Exp Biol Med 2008;233:901–13.

38. Danišovic L, Varga I, Polak S, et al. Comparison of in vitro chondrogenic potential of human mesenchymal stem cells derived from bone marrow and adipose tissue. Gen Physiol Biophys 2009;28:56–62.

39. Zhang J, Niu C, Ye L, et al. Identification of the haematopoietic stem cell niche and control of the niche size. Nature 2003;425:836–41.

40. Tumbar T, Guasch G, Greco V, et al. Defining the epithelial stem cell niche in skin. Science 2004;303:359–63.

41. Barker N, van Es JH, Kuipers J, et al. Identification of stem cells in small intestine and colon by marker gene Lgr5. Nature 2007;449:1003–8.
42. Kuang S, Kuroda K, Le Grand F, et al. Asymmetric self-renewal and commitment of satellite stem cells in muscle. Cell 2007;129:999–1010.
43. da Silva Meirelles L, Chagastelles PC, Nardi NB. Mesenchymal stem cells reside in virtually all post-natal organs and tissues. J Cell Sci 2006;119:2204–13.
44. Jones DL, Wagers AJ. No place like home: anatomy and function of the stem cell niche. Nat Rev Mol Cell Biol 2008;9:11–21.
45. Sacchetti B, Funari A, Michienzi S, et al. Self-renewing osteoprogenitors in bone marrow sinusoids can organize a hematopoietic microenvironment. Cell 2007; 131:324–36.
46. Nöth U, Osyczka AM, Tuli R, et al. Multilineage mesenchymal differentiation potential of human trabecular bone-derived cells. J Orthop Res 2002;20: 1060–9.
47. Sakaguchi Y, Sekiya I, Yagishita K, et al. Suspended cells from trabecular bone by collagenase digestion become virtually identical to mesenchymal stem cells obtained from marrow aspirates. Blood 2004;104:2728–35.
48. Zhu H, Guo Z, Jiang X, et al. A protocol for isolation and culture of mesenchymal stem cells from mouse compact bone. Nat Protoc 2010;5:550–60.
49. Suva D, Garavaglia G, Menetry J, et al. Non-hematopoietic human bone marrow contains long-lasting, pluripotent mesenchymal stem cells. J Cell Physiol 2004; 198:110–8.
50. Kopesky PW, Lee HY, Vanderploeg EJ, et al. Adult equine bone marrow stromal cells produce a cartilage-like ECM mechanically superior to animal-matched adult chondrocytes. Matrix Biol 2010;29:427–38.
51. Arnhold SJ, Goletz I, Klein H, et al. Isolation and characterization of bone marrow-derived equine mesenchymal stem cells. Am J Vet Res 2007;231: 1095–105.
52. Kasashima Y, Ueno T, Tomita A, et al. Optimisation of bone marrow aspiration from the equine sternum for the safe recovery of mesenchymal stem cells. Equine Vet J 2011;43:288–94.
53. Schnabel L, Lynch M, van der Meulen M, et al. Mesenchymal stem cells and insulin-like growth factor-I gene-enhanced mesenchymal stem cells improve structural aspects of healing in equine flexor digitorum superficialis tendons. J Orthop Res 2009;27(10):1392–8.
54. Wilke MM, Nydam DV, Nixon AJ. Enhanced early chondrogenesis in articular defects following arthroscopic mesenchymal stem cell implantation in an equine model. J Orthop Res 2007;25:913–25.
55. Frisbie DD, Kisiday JD, Kawcak CE, et al. Evaluation of adipose derived stromal vascular fraction or bone marrow derived mesenchymal stem cells for treatment of osteoarthritis. J Orthop Res 2009;27:1675–80.
56. Smith RK, Korda M, Blunn GW, et al. Isolation and implantation of autologous equine mesenchymal stem cells from bone marrow into the superficial digital flexor tendon as a potential novel treatment. Equine Vet J 2003;35:99–102.
57. Pacini S, Spinabella S, Trombi L, et al. Suspension of bone marrow–derived undifferentiated mesenchymal stromal cells for repair of superficial digital flexor tendon in race horses. Tissue Eng 2007;13:2949–55.
58. Godwin EE, Young NJ, Dudhia J, et al. Implantation of bone marrow-derived mesenchymal stem cells demonstrates improved outcome in horses with over-strain injury of the superficial digital flexor tendon. Equine Vet J 2011. DOI:10.1111/j.2042-3306.2011.00363.x. [Epub ahead of print].

59. Ferris DJ, Frisbie DD, Kisiday JD, et al. Clinical follow-up of horses treated with bone marrow derived mesenchymal stem cells for musculoskeletal lesions. Proc AAEP Ann Conv 2009;55:59.
60. Mambelli LI, Santos EJ, Fraza PJ, et al. Characterization of equine adipose tissue–derived progenitor cells before and after cryopreservation. Tissue Eng Part C Methods 2009;15:87–94.
61. da Silva Meirelles L, Sand TT, Harman RJ, et al. MSC frequency correlates with blood vessel density in equine adipose tissue. Tissue Eng Part A 2009;15:221–9.
62. Estes BT, Wu AW, Guilak F. Potent induction of chondrocytic differentiation of human adipose-derived adult stem cells by bone morphogenetic protein 6. Arthritis Rheum 2006;54:1222–32.
63. Gimble JM, Katz AJ, Bunnell BA. Adipose-derived stem cells for regenerative medicine. Circ Res 2007;100:1249–60.
64. Afizah H, Yang Z, Hui JH, et al. A comparison between the chondrogenic potential of human bone marrow stem cells (BMSCs) and adipose-derived stem cells (ADSCs) taken from the same donors. Tissue Eng 2007;13:659–66.
65. Huang JI, Kazmi N, Durbhakula MM, et al. Chondrogenic potential of progenitor cells derived from human bone marrow and adipose tissue: a patient-matched comparison. J Orthop Res 2000;5(23):1383–9.
66. Sakaguchi Y, Sekiya I, Yagishita K, et al. Comparison of human stem cells derived from various mesenchymal tissues. Arthritis Rheum 2005;52:2521–9.
67. Toupadakis CA, Wong A, Genetos DC, et al. Comparison of the osteogenic potential of equine mesenchymal stem cells from bone marrow, adipose tissue, umbilical cord blood, and umbilical cord tissue. Am J Vet Res 2010;71:1237–45.
68. Kisiday JD, Kopesky PW, Evans CH, et al. Evaluation of adult equine bone marrow- and adipose-derived progenitor cell chondrogenesis in hydrogel cultures. J Orthop Res 2008;26:322–31.
69. Vidal MA, Robinson SO, Lopez MJ, et al. Comparison of chondrogenic potential in equine mesenchymal stromal cells derived from adipose tissue and bone marrow. Vet Surg 2008;37:713–24.
70. Hennig T, Lorenz H, Thiel A, et al. Reduced chondrogenic potential of adipose tissue derived stromal cells correlates with an altered TGFβ receptor and BMP profile and is overcome by BMP-6. J Cell Physiol 2007;21:682–91.
71. Gonzalez-Rey E, Gonzalez MA, Varela N, et al. Human adipose-derived mesenchymal stem cells reduce inflammatory and T cell responses and induce regulatory T cells in vitro in rheumatoid arthritis. Ann Rheum Dis 2010;69:241–8.
72. Bochev I, Elmadjian G, Kyurkchiev D, et al. Mesenchymal stem cells from human bone marrow or adipose tissue differently modulate mitogen-stimulated B-cell immunoglobulin production in vitro. Cell Biol Int 2008;32:384–93.
73. English A, Jones EA, Corscadden D, et al. A comparative assessment of cartilage and joint fat pad as a potential source of cells for autologous therapy development in knee osteoarthritis. Rheumatology 2007;46:1676–83.
74. Petsa A, Gargani S, Felesakis A, et al. Effectiveness of protocol for the isolation of Wharton's Jelly stem cells in large-scale applications. In Vitro Cell Dev Biol Anim 2009;45:573–6.
75. Troyer DL, Weiss ML. Concise review: Wharton's Jelly-derived cells are a primitive stromal cell population. Stem Cells 2008;26:591–9.
76. Barachini S, Trombi L, Danti S, et al. Morpho-functional characterization of human mesenchymal stem cells from umbilical cord blood for potential uses in regenerative medicine. Stem Cells Dev 2009;18:293–305.

77. Bi Y, Ehirchiou D, Kilts TM, et al. Identification of tendon stem/progenitor cells and the role of the extracellular matrix in their niche. Nat Med 2007;13:1219–27.

78. Stewart AA, Barrett JG, Byron CR, et al. Comparison of equine tendon-, muscle-, and bone marrow-derived cells cultured on tendon matrix. Am J Vet Res 2009; 70:750–7.

79. Rui YF, Phil M, Lui PP, et al. Isolation and characterization of multipotent rat tendon-derived stem cells. Tissue Eng Part A 2010;16:1549–58.

80. Salingcarnboriboon R, Yoshitake H, Tsuji K, et al. Establishment of tendon-derived cell lines exhibiting pluripotent mesenchymal stem cell-like property. Exp Cell Res 2003;287:289–300.

81. Yoshimura H, Muneta T, Nimura A, et al. Comparison of rat mesenchymal stem cells derived from bone marrow, synovium, periosteum, adipose tissue, and muscle. Cell Tissue Res 2007;327:449–62.

82. Nishimura K, Solchaga LA, Caplan AI, et al. Chondroprogenitor cells of synovial tissue. Arthritis Rheum 1999;42:2631–7.

83. Pei M, He F, Chen D, et al. Synovium-derived stem cell-based chondrogenesis. Differentiation 2008;76:1044–56.

84. Shintani N, Hunziker EB. Chondrogenic differentiation of bovine synovium: bone morphogenetic proteins 2 and 7 and transforming growth factor β1 induce the formation of different types of cartilaginous tissue. Arthritis Rheum 2007;56: 1869–79.

85. De Bari C, Dell'Accio F, Tylzanowski P, et al. Multipotent mesenchymal stem cells from adult human synovial membrane. Arthritis Rheum 2001;44:1928–42.

86. Kurth T, Hedbom E, Shintani N, et al. Chondrogenic potential of human synovial mesenchymal stem cells in alginate. Osteoarthritis Cartilage 2007;15:1178–89.

87. Arufe MC, De la Fuente A, Fuentes-Boquete I, et al. Differentiation of Synovial CD-105þ human mesenchymal stem cells into chondrocyte-like cells through spheroid formation. J Cell Biochem 2009;108:145–55.

88. Ichinose S, Muneta T, Koga H, et al. Morphological differences during in vitro chondrogenesis of bone marrow-, synovium-MSCs, and chondrocytes. Lab Invest 2010;90:210–21.

89. Dowthwaite GP, Bishop JC, Redman SN, et al. The surface of articular cartilage contains a progenitor cell population. J Cell Sci 2003;117:889–97.

90. Alsalameh S, Amin R, Gemba T, et al. Identification of mesenchymal progenitor cells in normal and osteoarthritic human articular cartilage. Arthritis Rheum 2004;50:1522–32.

91. Koga H, Muneta T, Ju YJ, et al. Synovial stem cells are regionally specified according to local microenvironments after implantation for cartilage regeneration. Stem Cells 2007;25:689–96.

92. Chen Y, Kuykendall TD, Caporali E, et al. Cells in equine synovial fluid exhibit chondrogenic capacity without evidence of an endochondral phenotype. Trans Orthop Res Soc 2009;34:937.

93. Kuznetsov SA, Mankani MH, Gronthos S, et al. Circulating skeletal stem cells. J Cell Biol 2001;153:1133–9.

94. Kuznetsov SA, Mankani MH, Leet AI, et al. Circulating connective tissue precursors: extreme rarity in humans and chondrogenic potential in guinea pigs. Stem Cells 2007;25:1830–9.

95. Tondreau T, Nathalie Meuleman N, Alain Delforge A. Mesenchymal stem cells derived from CD133-positive cells in mobilized peripheral blood and cord blood: proliferation, Oct4 expression, and plasticity. Stem Cells 2005;23: 1105–12.

96. Giovannini S, Brehm W, Mainil-Varlet P, et al. Multilineage differentiation potential of equine blood-derived fibroblast-like cells. Differentiation 2008;76:118–29.

97. Koerner J, Nesic D, Romero JD, et al. Equine peripheral blood-derived progenitors in comparison to bone marrow-derived mesenchymal stem cells. Stem Cells 2006;24:1613–9.

98. Ahern BJ, Schaer TP, Shawn P, et al. Evaluation of equine peripheral blood apheresis product, bone marrow, and adipose tissue as sources of mesenchymal stem cells and their differentiation potential. Am J Vet Res 2011;72: 127–33.

99. Kasten P, Beyen I, Egermann M, et al. Instant stem cell therapy: characterization and concentration of human mesenchymal stem cells in vitro. Eur Cell Mater 2008;16:47–55.

100. Nishimoto S, Oyama T, Matsuda K. Simultaneous concentration of platelets and marrow cells: a simple and useful technique to obtain source cells and growth factors for regenerative medicine. Wound Repair Regen 2007;15:156–62.

101. Di Bella C, Barbara Dozza B, Frisoni T, et al. Injection of demineralized bone matrix with bone marrow concentrate improves healing in unicameral bone cyst. Clin Orthop Relat Res 2010;468:3047–55.

102. Jäger M, Herten M, Fochtmann U, et al. Bridging the gap: bone marrow aspiration concentrate reduces autologous bone grafting in osseous defects. J Orthop Res 2010;29:173–80.

103. Hernigou P, Poignard A, Beaujean F, et al. Percutaneous autologous bone-marrow grafting for nonunions: influence of the number and concentration of progenitor cells. J Bone Joint Surg Am 2005;87:1430–7.

104. Vadalá G, Di Martino A, Tirindelli MC, et al. Use of autologous bone marrow cells concentrate enriched with platelet-rich fibrin on corticocancellous bone allograft for posterolateral multilevel cervical fusion. J Tissue Eng Regen Med 2008;2: 515–20.

105. Yoshioka T, Mishima H, Akaogi H, et al. Concentrated autologous bone marrow aspirate transplantation treatment for corticosteroid-induced osteonecrosis of the femoral head in systemic lupus erythematosus. Int Orthop 2011;35:823–9.

106. Fortier LA, Potter HG, Rickey EJ, et al. Concentrated bone marrow aspirate improves full-thickness cartilage repair compared with microfracture in the equine model. J Bone Joint Surg Am 2010;92:1927–37.

107. Chang F, Ishii T, Yanai T, et al. Repair of large full-thickness articular cartilage defects by transplantation of autologous uncultured bone-marrow-derived mononuclear cells. J Orthop Res 2008;26:18–26.

108. Crovace A, Lacitignola L, Rossi G, et al. Histological and immunohistochemical evaluation of autologous cultured bone marrow mesenchymal stem cells and bone marrow mononucleated cells in collagenase-induced tendinitis of equine superficial digital flexor tendon. Vet Med Int 2010;2010:250978.

109. Varma MJ, Breuls RG, Schouten TE, et al. Phenotypical and functional characterization of freshly isolated adipose tissue-derived stem cells. Stem Cells Dev 2007;16:91–104.

110. Nixon AJ, Dahlgren LA, Haupt JL, et al. Effect of adipose-derived nucleated cell fractions on tendon repair in horses with collagenase-induced tendinitis. Am J Vet Res 2008;69:928–37.

111. Vet-Stem Inc. Available at: http://vet-stem.com/equine/casestudies.php. Accessed July 14, 2011.

112. Caplan AI. Mesenchymal stem cells: cell-based reconstructive therapy in orthopedics. Tissue Eng 2005;11:1198–211.

113. Karlsson C, Brantsing C, Svensson T, et al. Differentiation of human mesenchymal stem cells and articular chondrocytes: analysis of chondrogenic potential and expression pattern of differentiation-related transcription factors. J Orthop Res 2007;25:152–63.
114. Mienaltowski MJ, Huang L, Frisbie DD, et al. Transcriptional profiling differences for articular cartilage and repair tissue in equine joint surface lesions. BMC Med Genomics 2009;2:60.
115. De Bari C, Dell'Accio F, Luyten FP. Failure of in vitro–differentiated mesenchymal stem cells from the synovial membrane to form ectopic stable cartilage in vivo. Arthritis Rheum 2004;50:142–50.
116. Stewart MC, Saunders KM, Burton-Wurster N, et al. Phenotypic stability of articular chondrocytes *in vitro*: the effects of culture models, BMP-2 and serum supplementation. J Bone Miner Res 2000;15:166–74.
117. Quintavallaa J, Uziel-Fusia S, Yin J, et al. Fluorescently labeled mesenchymal stem cells (MSCs) maintain multilineage potential and can be detected following implantation into articular cartilage defects. Biomaterials 2002;23:109–19.
118. Guest DJ, Smith MR, Allen WR. Equine embryonic stem-like cells and mesenchymal stromal cells have different survival rates and migration patterns following their injection into damaged superficial digital flexor tendon. Equine Vet J 2010;42:636–42.
119. Murphy JM, Fink DJ, Hunziker EB, et al. Stem cell therapy in a caprine model of osteoarthritis. Arthritis Rheum 2003;48:3464–74.
120. Hill CE, Proschel C, Noble M, et al. Acute transplantation of glial-restricted precursor cells into spinal cord contusion injuries: survival, differentiation, and effects on lesion environment and axonal regeneration. Exp Neurol 2004;190:289–310.
121. Kuh SU, Cho YE, Yoon DH, et al. Functional recovery after human umbilical cord blood cells transplantation with brain-derived neutrophic factor into the spinal cord injured rat. Acta Neurochir (Wien) 2005;147:985–92.
122. Kuraitis D, Ruel M, Suuronen EJ. Mesenchymal stem cells for cardiovascular regeneration. Cardiovasc Drugs Ther 2011;25(4):349–62.
123. Caplan AI, Dennis JE. Mesenchymal stem cells as trophic mediators. J Cell Biochem 2006;98:1076–84.
124. Haynesworth SE, Baber MA, Caplan AI. Cytokine expression by human marrow-derived mesenchymal progenitor cells in vitro: effects of dexamethasone and IL-1 alpha. J Cell Physiol 1996;166:585–92.
125. Phinney DG, Hill K, Michelson C, et al. Biological activities encoded by the murine mesenchymal stem cell transcriptome provide a basis for their developmental potential and broad therapeutic efficacy. Stem Cells 2006;24:186–98.
126. Silva GV, Litovsky S, Assad JA, et al. Mesenchymal stem cells differentiate into an endothelial phenotype, enhance vascular density, and improve heart function in a canine chronic ischemia model. Circulation 2005;111:150–6.
127. Tang J, Xie Q, Pan G, et al. Mesenchymal stem cells participate in angiogenesis and improve heart function in rat model of myocardial ischemia with reperfusion. Eur J Cardiothorac Surg 2006;30:353–61.
128. Sadat S, Gehmert S, Song YH, et al. The cardioprotective effect of mesenchymal stem cells is mediated by IGF-I and VEGF. Biochem Biophys Res Commun 2007;363:674–9.
129. Amado LC, Saliaris AP, Schuleri KH, et al. Cardiac repair with intramyocardial injection of allogeneic mesenchymal stem cells after myocardial infarction. Proc Natl Acad Sci U S A 2005;102:11474–9.

130. Li Q, Turdi S, Thomas DP, et al. Intra-myocardial delivery of mesenchymal stem cells ameliorates left ventricular and cardiomyocyte contractile dysfunction following myocardial infarction. Toxicol Lett 2010;195:119–26.

131. Gnecchi M, He H, Noiseux N, et al. Evidence supporting paracrine hypothesis for Akt-modified mesenchymal stem cell-mediated cardiac protection and functional improvement. FASEB J 2006;20:661–9.

132. Shabbir A, Zisa D, Suzuki G, et al. Heart failure therapy mediated by the trophic activities of bone marrow mesenchymal stem cells: a noninvasive therapeutic regimen. Am J Physiol Heart Circ Physiol 2009;296:H1888–97.

133. Li Y, Chen J, Zhang C, et al. Gliosis and brain remodeling after treatment of stroke in rats with marrow stromal cells. Glia 2005;49:407–17.

134. Harms KM, Li L, Cunningham LA. Murine neural stem/progenitor cells protect neurons against ischemia by HIF-1α–regulated VEGF signaling. PLoS One 2010;5:e9767. DOI:10.1371/journal.pone.0009767.

135. Syková E, Jendelová P, Urdzíková L, et al. Bone marrow stem cells and polymer hydrogels—two strategies for spinal cord injury repair. Cell Mol Neurobiol 2006;26:1113–29.

136. Wei X, Zhao L, Zhong J, et al. Adipose stromal cells-secreted neuroprotective media against neuronal apoptosis. Neurosci Lett 2009;462:76–9.

137. Lee RH, Pulin AA, Seo MJ, et al. Intravenous hMSCs improve myocardial infarction in mice because cells embolized in lung are activated to secrete the anti-inflammatory protein TSG-6. Cell Stem Cell 2009;5:54–63.

138. Ryan JM, Barry F, Murphy JM, et al. Interferon-γ does not break, but promotes the immunosuppressive capacity of adult human mesenchymal stem cells. Clin Exp Immunol 2007;149:353–63.

139. Shi Y, Hu G, Su J, et al. Mesenchymal stem cells: a new strategy for immunosuppression and tissue repair. Cell Res 2010;20:510–8.

140. Zheng ZH, Li XY, Ding J, et al. Allogeneic mesenchymal stem cell and mesenchymal stem cell-differentiated chondrocyte suppress the responses of type II collagen-reactive T cells in rheumatoid arthritis. Rheumatology 2008;47:22–30.

Collection and Propagation Methods for Mesenchymal Stromal Cells

Sarah E. Taylor, BVM&S, MSc, PhD, Cert ES(Orth), MRCVS[a],*,
Peter D. Clegg, MA, Vet MB, PhD[b]

KEYWORDS

- Mesenchymal stromal cell • Progenitor cell • Stem cell
- Differentiation • Equine

Mesenchymal stromal cells (MSC) are derived from adult mesenchymal tissues and have the ability to undergo differentiation into bone, cartilage, and fat. MSC were originally collected from the bone marrow stroma,[1] but it has since been found that they exist in many tissues.[1–4] The most commonly used sources of MSC in the clinical setting are bone marrow, adipose tissue, and umbilical cord blood. The production of MSC for clinical use must adhere to good manufacturing practice to ensure delivery of a safe, reproducible, and efficient "cell therapy."[5] Many isolation and culture methods have been described, with variable differentiation protocols and few comparative assessments to guide selection of optimal protocols. A consensus on the definition and properties of MSC after in vitro expansion has recently been reached for human MSC by the International Society for Cellular Therapy[6]: ex vivo adherence to tissue culture plastic, multilineage differentiation, and a specific immunophenotype. This definition has not yet been specifically applied to equine MSC even though many of these criteria have been demonstrated. A uniform protocol to characterize equine MSC has recently been proposed, to introduce consistency across the equine stem cell research field.[4] This article reviews the published techniques for collection and propagation of equine MSC, focusing on bone marrow–derived and adipose-derived cells. Where appropriate, comparative studies in humans and other species are also referred to.

The authors have nothing to disclose.
[a] Department of Veterinary Clinical Sciences, University of Edinburgh, Dick Vet Equine Hospital, Easter Bush Vet Centre, Roslin, Midlothian, EH25 9RG, UK
[b] Department of Musculoskeletal Biology, University of Liverpool, Leahurst Campus, Chester High Road, Neston, Cheshire, CH64 7TE, UK
* Corresponding author.
E-mail address: Sarah.e.taylor@ed.ac.uk

Vet Clin Equine 27 (2011) 263–274
doi:10.1016/j.cveq.2011.05.003
0749-0739/11/$ – see front matter © 2011 Elsevier Inc. All rights reserved.

vetequine.theclinics.com

COLLECTION TECHNIQUES FOR BONE MARROW–DERIVED MSC

The sternum is the most commonly used site for aspiration of equine bone marrow–derived MSC (BM-MSC), as described by Smith and colleagues.[7] Although most veterinarians believe sternal bone marrow aspiration to be a relatively innocuous procedure, there have been case reports of iatrogenic cardiac puncture[8] and nonfatal pneumopericardium.[9] A recent article has described the fifth sternebra to be the safest site for aspiration, as it has the largest dorsoventral span and is cranial to the apex of the heart (**Fig. 1**).[10] In brief, the horse is sedated with an α2-agonist (detomidine, 10 μg/kg) with or without an opiate (butorphanol, 20 μg/kg); a 10 × 10 cm^2 area over the sternum is clipped and saturated with warm water before application of ultrasound coupling gel just caudal to the elbow. The sternebrae are palpated and then ultrasonographically imaged using a 10-MHz linear probe to identify two sternebrae and the intersternebral space (**Fig. 2**). If need be, the site is identified by use of a sterile marker pen.

The site is then cleaned and aseptically prepared. Local analgesia is injected into the site (mepivicaine, 5 mL) using a 21-gaugeG 1.5-inch (38.1 mm) needle. A No. 11 scalpel blade is used to make a stab incision over the sternebra. A 12-gauge Jamshidi needle is introduced into the stab incision and advanced until contact with cortical bone is made. The Jamshidi needle is then advanced 1.5 cm through the cortical bone of the sternebra and into the medullary cavity. It is prudent to place a finger 2 cm from the sharp end of the needle while it is being rotated and advanced through cortical bone, to act as a "stop" and prevent intrathoracic penetration. A 20-mL syringe preloaded with 5000 IU of heparin is connected to the Jamshidi needle and 10 to 15 mL of bone marrow is aspirated (**Fig. 3**). The aspirated sample is mixed by inverting several times and transferred aseptically to a 20-mL sterile falcon tube before immediate density gradient centrifugation (see later discussion).

Alternative sites for bone marrow aspiration include the tuber coxae, tibia, and humerus. Aspiration from the tuber coxae is performed from the ventral third of the iliac wing, approximately 4 cm axial to the tuber coxae.[11] The Jamshidi needle is angled slightly caudally, in the direction of the contralateral coxfemoral joint (**Fig. 4**).

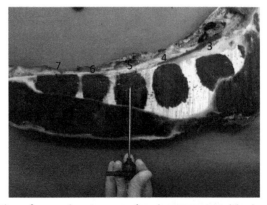

Fig. 1. Sagittal section of an equine sternum, showing correct positioning of a Jamshidi needle within the marrow cavity of the fifth sternebrae. (*Courtesy of* Matthew C. Stewart, BVSc, PhD and Allison A. Stewart, DVM, MS, Department of Veterinary Clinical Medicine, College of Veterinary Medicine, University of Illinois, USA.)

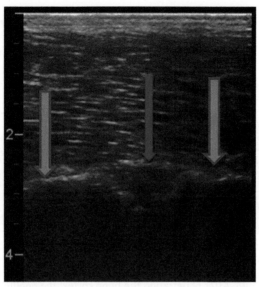

Fig. 2. Ultrasonogram of two equine sternebrae (*blue arrows*) and the intersternebral space (*red arrow*). The horse's ventral midline is at the top of the image. The intersternebral space should be avoided when aspirating bone marrow.

COLLECTION TECHNIQUES FOR ADIPOSE-DERIVED MSC

Adipose tissue is most commonly harvested from the tail head of horses under standing sedation and local anesthesia.[11–13] The same sedation protocol as used for BM-MSC aspiration can be used. Local anesthesia is provided by a line block using 10 to 20 mL of 1% lidocaine or equivalent. A 10-cm linear incision is made lateral to the tail head and 9 to 10 g of adipose tissue is harvested using tissue forceps,[11] and placed in a sterile container. The subcutaneous tissue is closed with polyglactin 910 in a simple continuous pattern, and the skin is closed with staples.[11] Alternatively, adipose tissue can be harvested from the area over the dorsal gluteal muscles. The skin and subcutaneous tissues are desensitized using an inverted L-block. A 10- to 15-cm incision is made parallel and about 15 cm abaxial to the vertebral column.

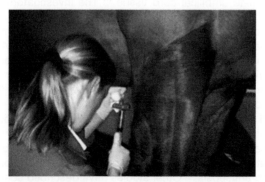

Fig. 3. Sternal bone marrow aspiration from an adult horse using a 12-gauge Jamshidi needle. Note the position of the aspiration site, relative to the forelimb of the horse.

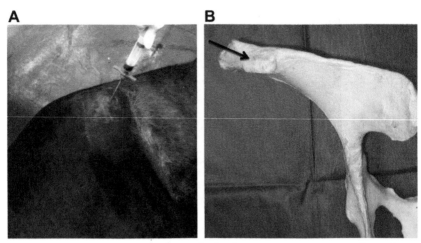

Fig. 4. (*A*) Positioning of a Jamshidi needle for bone marrow aspiration from the tuber coxae. The needle is directed axially and caudally after insertion. (*B*) A skeletal preparation of the ilium, showing the direction required to position the needle within the marrow cavity of the ileal wing (*arrow*). After penetrating the bone cortex, the needle should be directed toward the contralateral coxofemoral joint. (*Courtesy of* Allison A. Stewart, DVM, MS and Eric R. Carlson, DVM, Department of Veterinary Clinical Medicine, College of Veterinary Medicine, University of Illinois, USA.)

Adipose tissue (about 15 mL) is harvested over the superficial gluteal fascia for adipose tissue MSC (AT-MSC) isolation. The skin incision is apposed with nylon suture material.[14,15] The number of AT-MSC harvested from fat tissue has been correlated with blood vessel density in one study.[16]

COLLECTION TECHNIQUES FOR UMBILICAL CORD–DERIVED MSC

MSC were first derived from umbilical cord blood collected before the umbilical cord spontaneously broke via venipuncture of the umbilical vein.[17] The sample was collected using a 16-gauge needle attached to a 450-mL blood collection bag containing citrate phosphate dextrose adenine (CPDA) as the anticoagulant. More recently, a detailed protocol has been described for the collection of equine umbilical cord blood and equine umbilical cord tissue.[18] The investigators describe aseptic preparation of the umbilical cord with chlorhexidine followed by isopropyl alcohol, and the use of a cable tie placed 6 to 8 cm from the foal's umbilicus. Sampling into a collection bag or a collection syringe preloaded with CPDA was compared; no significant differences were identified between the volumes collected with each system (141 mL and 122 mL, respectively). Blood collected using the syringe technique was transferred to a 250-mL collection bag and kept at 4°C for transportation to the laboratory to minimize bacterial infection.[18]

Equine umbilical cord tissue can be collected by placing a second cable tie 10 cm away from the initial cable tie (placed 6–8 cm from the foal's umbilicus) and then cutting the umbilical cord with scissors. The midsection of the umbilical cord is then rinsed with tap water to remove gross contamination and then submerged in 0.05% chlorhexidine to aid antisepsis.[18] Other studies have described soaking the umbilical cord tissue in medium containing penicillin/streptomycin and amphotericin.[11]

ISOLATION AND IN VITRO CULTURE OF BONE MARROW–DERIVED MSC

The density of MSC in bone marrow is very low (0.01%–0.001%); therefore, techniques to expand cell numbers in vitro have been developed. Several techniques for the isolation of MSC from bone marrow aspirates have been described. Neat bone marrow can be transferred to tissue culture flasks in a tissue culture hood and cultured with growth medium (Dulbecco's modified Eagle's medium [DMEM], 10% fetal calf serum, penicillin, and streptomycin: approximately 1 mL of bone marrow added to a T75 tissue culture flask containing 18 mL of medium). Alternatively, bone marrow can be centrifuged at 1000 × *g* for 15 minutes and the cell pellet resuspended in medium before seeding.[19] This "classic" technique used to select bone marrow MSC is based on their ability to adhere to tissue culture plastic.[19,20]

More commonly, the bone marrow aspirate is placed on a density gradient solution and the mononuclear cell fraction is separated by centrifugation, prior to aspiration and culture. Density gradient separation separates the mononuclear cell fraction from the red blood cells, granulocytes, platelets, and immature precursors in the initial aspirate. Mononuclear cells have a density of 1.073 g/dL; therefore, they are commonly isolated in a ring of density gradient centrifugation (1.077 g/dL Ficoll). The other density gradient solution reported for equine MSC is Percoll, which has a density of 1.084 g/dL. There are many articles in the equine literature that use either the Ficoll[7,20,21] density gradient solution or the Percoll[19,22] density gradient solution for mononuclear cell fractionation. A recent article highlighted possible differences between the two density gradient solutions and suggested that Percoll may have better MSC yield and self-renewal, but these differences were seen only in primary cultures. No difference in osteogenic and chondrogenic potential was seen in cell populations isolated by the two density gradient solutions or in comparison with cells not subject to density gradient separation. The investigators did suggest that Percoll may minimize culture time.[19] The aspirated mononuclear fraction is collected and plated into tissue culture flasks at $1–25 \times 10^3$ MSC/cm^2. The authors use an initial plating density of 5×10^3 MSC/cm^2, as lower plating densities allow greater numbers of adherent cells.[23]

MSC are usually expanded in growth medium containing 10% fetal bovine serum (FBS) to provide essential proteins for cellular adhesion and growth. Growth in serum-free medium slows cell proliferation, prolongs the time in culture, and promotes an early progenitor cell phenotype with increased expression of embryonic stem cell genes.[5] Culture of equine BM-MSC with autologous serum instead of FBS also significantly slows growth.[11] Antibiotics and antifungal agents are commonly added to the growth medium (100 U/mL penicillin, 100 μg/mL streptomycin, and 2.5 μg/mL amphotericin B, respectively). The specific composition of growth medium varies in different published studies; the most frequently used are DMEM[10,19] and α-MEM.[20] A technical study using human BM-MSC found α-MEM + Glutamax + 10% FBS and α-MEM +L-glutamine + 10% FBS allowed the most rapid cell expansion while maintaining multipotent characteristics.[23] MSC are allowed to adhere for 4 days before the initial media change. Thereafter, the medium is usually changed every 2 to 3 days during cell expansion. Once MSC are confluent (**Fig. 5**), the cells are released from the flask by trypsin digestion and passaged. If cells are allowed to become overconfluent they can become senescent or may begin to differentiate from their uncommitted status.

The adherent cells are released by removing growth medium and then washing the cell layer with Hanks' Balanced Salt Solution to remove any traces of FBS, as FBS can inactivate trypsin. For a T75 flask, approximately 4 mL of 0.05% trypsin-EDTA (ethylenediamine tetra-acetic acid) will cover the bottom of the flask and effect cell release.

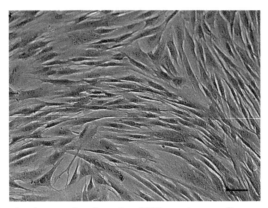

Fig. 5. Phase-contrast micrograph of equine MSC nearing confluence. Scale bar: 10 μm. (*Courtesy of* Allison A. Stewart, DVM, MS, Department of Veterinary Clinical Medicine, College of Veterinary Medicine, University of Illinois, USA.)

The flask containing trypsin-EDTA is placed at 37°C for 5 to 7 minutes. MSC are more sensitive to trypsin-EDTA than other cell types and therefore, to increase homogeneity at earlier passages, trypsinization should never exceed 5 to 6 minutes at 37°C.[23] Once cellular detachment has been observed under the microscope, the trypsin-EDTA solution is neutralized with growth medium containing 10% FCS (67 μl/cm², 5 ml/T75 culture flask). The cells are then pipetted up and down repeatedly to produce a single cell suspension and transferred to a sterile Falcon tube. The cell suspension is centrifuged at 1100 rpm for 4 minutes and the cell pellet is resuspended in an appropriate volume of cell culture medium following cell counting.

ISOLATION AND IN VITRO CULTURE OF ADIPOSE-DERIVED MSC

Adipose tissue is minced with a surgical blade, washed, and briefly agitated with an equal volume of phosphate-buffered saline (PBS) solution to promote separation into two phases. The upper phase consists of minced and washed adipose tissue and the lower phase contains hematopoietic cells suspended in PBS. The lower phase is discarded. The adipose tissue is digested in an equal volume of PBS solution containing 1% bovine serum albumin and 0.1% collagenase on an orbital shaker, shaking continuously for 50 minutes at 37°C. To complete stromal cell separation from adipocytes, the sample is briefly and vigorously agitated before being centrifuged at $260 \times g$ for 5 minutes. The supernatant is discarded and the cell pellet containing the nucleated cells including AT-MSC is then cultured in DMEM-Ham's F12 containing 10% FBS, penicillin/streptomycin.[14] Addition of basic fibroblast growth factor has been shown to enhance the proliferation rate of equine AT-MSC and BM-MSC while maintaining their differentiation potential.[24]

ISOLATION AND IN VITRO CULTURE OF UMBILICAL CORD–DERIVED MSC

Equine umbilical cord–derived MSC (UC-MSC) have been successfully cultured in several laboratories.[11,17,25,26] Consistent and reproducible isolation of UC-MSC has not been reported in any species, and the highest reported isolation percentage on selected cord blood samples is 63%.[26] The mononuclear cell fraction of equine umbilical cord blood has been isolated using 1.077 g/dL Ficoll and PrepaCyte-EQ medium

(BioE Inc, St Paul, MN, USA).[17,26] Superior isolation was reported with PrepaCyte-EQ medium.[26]

ASSAYS OF MSC CHARACTERISTICS AND ACTIVITIES
Self-Renewal and Clonogenicity (Colony-Forming Unit Assay)

A colony-forming unit (CFU) assay measures a cell population's or individual cell's capacity for self-renewal. In both cases, each colony is derived from the proliferation of a single cell.[1,27] The best way to carry out this assay is by single cell seeding after fluorescence-activated cell sorting. A simpler way to perform this assay is to plate the adherent MSC at very low density (18 cells/cm^2). Practically this can be done using 6-well tissue culture plates and plating cells at 185 cells/well. Cells are then cultured in growth media for 10 days with media changes every 3 to 4 days until colonies of approximately 50 cells form (**Fig. 6**). Colonies are then fixed in 70% ethanol and stained with 0.1% methylene blue, and counted. The number of colonies present reflects self-renewal potential of the initial cell population. The mean rate of equine BM-MSC colony formation demonstrated by one group was 27,[20] whereas other workers have demonstrated between 3 and 65 colonies per 9-cm diameter dish, dependent on isolation protocol and cell seeding density.[19]

It has recently been demonstrated that equine BM-MSC reach senescence more rapidly than AT-MSC or UC-MSC. BM-MSC become senescent after 30 population doublings compared with 60 to 80 population doublings for AT-MSC and UC-MSC.[28]

In Vitro Differentiation of MSC

Cellular differentiation refers to modifications in gene expression and metabolism that constitute a change in phenotype (cell shape, membrane potential, and metabolic activity). Multilineage differentiation is one of the minimum MSC criteria defined by the International Society for Cellular Therapy.[6] The 3 most established differentiation pathways for equine MSC destined for musculoskeletal use are the chondrogenic, osteogenic, and adipogenic lineages. Trilineage differentiation was first demonstrated for human BM-MSC.[29] Subsequently, there have been several adjustments and variations to the specific biochemical factors needed to effect in vitro differentiation, resulting in numerous protocols with only subtle differences. One difference between protocols is whether the MSC are plated at low density to form CFUs before induction

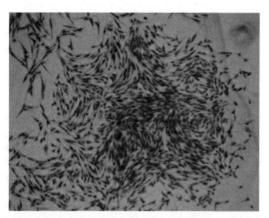

Fig. 6. Phase-contrast image of an equine MSC colony-forming unit stained with methylene blue.

medium is added. This step prolongs the culture time but may enhance differentiation. Certain differences in differentiation potential have been observed. For example, equine AT-MSC show reduced osteogenic capacity compared with BM-MSC.[13] Verification of differentiation is best performed using histologic assessment in conjunction with immune-phenotypic characterization and lineage-specific transcriptional profiling.

Osteogenic differentiation

Induction medium for osteogenesis requires the addition of 10 mmol/L β-glycerophosphate, 50 µg/mL ascorbic acid, and 20 nmol/L dexamethasone to standard MSC growth medium. The medium is changed every 2 to 3 days for 3 weeks until nodules can be detected under phase-contrast microscopy (see **Fig. 5**). Osteogenic differentiation can be identified by several methods: Alizarin Red[8,21] staining for calcium deposits; Von Kossa[20] staining to identify phosphate salts, or 5-bromo-4-chloro-indolyl phosphate nitroblue tetrazolium for detection of alkaline phosphatase activity.[20] Caution is advisable when using the Von Kossa protocol, as the silver ions react with phosphate and can produce false-positive areas of black staining. Genes that indicate osteogenic commitment include the transcription factor Cbfa1 (Runx2), bone sialoprotein (BSP), osteopontin (SPP1), and osteoprotegrin (OPN), all markers of early osteoblasts. Osteocalcin is a noncollagenous protein specific for late osteoblasts. Equine BM-MSC have demonstrated increased osteogenic potential when compared with AT-MSC.[13]

Chondrogenic differentiation

Chondrogenic differentiation is usually performed in cell pellets; aliquots of 500,000 cells/pellet are centrifuged at 1200 rpm for 5 minutes in 15 mL conical tubes. Pellets are cultured in the conical tubes for 2 weeks in serum-free chondrogenic differentiation medium (DMEM) containing 0.5 µg/mL of insulin-transferrin-sodium selenite media supplement (ITS), 10 nM dexamethasone, 10 ng/mL transforming growth factor β1, 50 ng/mL ascorbic acid, and 50 mg/mL bovine serum albumin.[30] Differentiation medium is changed every 3 to 4 days. The weight of the cell pellet is recorded at the end of the culture period, and some pellets are collected for histology and stained for sulfated glycosaminoglycans using Safranin-O. Toluidine blue and Alcian blue can also be used to stain proteoglycans. Gene expression analysis for chondrogenic differentiation should include the transcription factor SOX9 and the matrix components collagen type II (COL2A1) and aggrecan (AGC1), as well as the hypertrophic marker collagen type X (COL10A1).[4]

Equine AT-MSC have reduced chondrogenic potential compared with BM-MSC in pellet culture.[14] In addition, AT-MSC have reduced chondrogenic potential in hydrogel culture compared with equine BM-MSC, as demonstrated by reduced gene expression and protein deposition of collagen type II in AT-MSC cultures.[12]

Adipogenic differentiation

Adipogenic differentiation of equine MSC has slightly different requirements compared with human MSC, in that rabbit serum needs to be added to the culture medium in addition to FBS.[17,18,21,31,32] Adipogenesis is associated with elevation of cyclic adenosine monophosphate (cAMP), which can be stimulated in vitro via the phosphodiesterase inhibitor, isobutylmethylxanthine (IBMX). Adipogenic induction medium consists of DMEM-Ham's F12, 3% FBS, 175 µmol/L pantothenate, 33 µmol/L biotin, 1 µmol/L insulin, 1 µmol/L dexamethasone, 0.5 mmol/L IBMX, 5 µmol/L rosiglitazone (Avandia; Glaxo Smith Kline, Cidra, Puerto Rico), and 5% rabbit serum.[32] Subconfluent MSC are exposed to the adipogenic induction medium for 3 days and thereafter the same medium without IBMX and Avandia to maintain adipocyte cell culture. Adipogenic differentiation can be identified histologically using Oil Red O to stain for neutral lipid formation. Upregulation of lipoprotein lipase and peroxisome proliferator-activated receptor γ mRNA expression indicates adipogenic differentiation.

Cryopreservation

Cryopreservation of MSC can be safely performed with minimal effects on cell viability and differentiation capabilities.[19,24,33] Osteogenic, chondrogenic, and adipogenic differentiation is also preserved for equine AT-MSC after cryopreservation.[34] Freezing of cells is performed in cell preservation fluid containing 10% dimethylsulfoxide (DMSO) and FBS. Following tryptic release of monolayer cells, the cell pellet is resuspended in cryopreservation medium (1×10^6 cells/mL) (DMEM + 10% FBS and 10% DMSO). The cells are frozen down in 1-mL aliquots in 1.5-mL cryogenic vials at a rate of 1°C decrease in temperature per minute, and stored at −80°C. This slow progressive decrease in temperature can be achieved using a freezing box containing room-temperature isopropyl ethanol. Cells that had been stored at −80°C should be rapidly thawed by placing them at 37°C for 2 to 3 minutes. The cells are then transferred to a T75 culture flask and 19 mL of warm (37°C) growth medium added.

CD Marker Characterization

"Cluster of differentiation" (CD) markers are cell surface markers used to characterize cell types. No single CD marker has been found to definitively identify MSC to date. To characterize a homogeneous population, a combination of markers should therefore be used. The International Society for Cellular Therapy states that human MSC all express CD73, CD90, and CD105 but do not express CD14, CD11b, CD34, CD45, CD79, CD19, or major histocompatibility complex (MHC)-II.[5] In addition to those markers reported by the International Society for Cellular Therapy, other workers report the expression of CD29, CD44, CD106, and CD166 on human MSC.[29] Surface marker characterization of equine MSC is lacking, with only a handful of published reports.[24,25,35–37] This lack of characterization may in part be due to the limited availability of species-specific or cross-reacting monoclonal antibodies for the horse.[38,39] The lack of cross-reactivity highlights the need for reliable positive and negative controls when performing immunohistochemistry or flow cytometry on equine MSC. Despite the difficulties with cross-reactivity, a recommendation for CD marker expression in equine MSC has been made: equine MSC should express CD29, CD44, and CD90, and lack expression of CD14, CD79, and MHC-II.[4]

COMPLICATIONS ASSOCIATED WITH IN VITRO MANAGEMENT OF CELL ISOLATION

Any cell culture system can be subject to bacterial or fungal contamination. This contamination is usually easily identified as cells begin to grow more slowly, culture medium changes from red to orange/yellow color, and fungal hyphae or bacteria are readily identified under phase-contrast microscopy. Once cells become infected, they must be discarded and are obviously unsuitable for clinical use.

Maintaining a homogeneous cell population is difficult when culturing MSC, but this can be encouraged by following simple cell culture protocols. MSC are very sensitive to trypsin, and prewarmed trypsin-EDTA should be applied for no longer than 5 to 7 minutes at 37°C to reduce the release of monocytes.[5,32] Direct cell-to-cell contact can promote spontaneous differentiation if cells are allowed to become overconfluent, and cells should be split at about 80% confluence.

MAINTENANCE OF FACILITIES AND QUALITY CONTROL

Culture of MSC should involve proper use of a laminar flow tissue culture hood that is well maintained and sterilized with isopropyl alcohol before and after use. All media should be made fresh and nonsterile media components should be sterilized by filtration through a 0.6-μm filter. The addition of antibiotics and antifungal agents can help reduce the frequency of infections but cannot replace good sterile technique when handling the specimens and cell cultures. Incubators are usually maintained in a humidified environment through means of a water bath that should be regularly checked and cleaned.

Quality-control polymerase chain reaction (PCR) assays are becoming available for human MSC to verify performance of stem cell media products.[40] This development may lead to the expansion of the criteria for identifying MSC.

SUMMARY

Equine MSC are freely available to the practitioner, yet there remains no consensus as to which cell types are the optimal sources to treat specific musculoskeletal conditions. Preliminary work suggests equine AT-MSC have inferior chondrogenic and osteogenic potential in vitro, but it is uncertain how this transfers to the clinical setting. Equine MSC research should aim to establish a uniform protocol for the characterization of MSC to allow implementation of quality control and also to improve the ability to compare research outcomes from different laboratories.

REFERENCES

1. Friedenstein AJ, Deriglasova UF, Kulagina NN, et al. Precursors for fibroblasts in different populations of hematopoietic cells as detected by the in vitro colony assay method. Exp Hematol 1974;2(2):83–92.
2. Taylor SE, Smith RK, Clegg PD. Mesenchymal stem cell therapy in equine musculoskeletal disease: scientific fact or clinical fiction? Equine Vet J 2007;39(2): 172–80.
3. Crisan M, Yap S, Casteilla L, et al. A perivascular origin for mesenchymal stem cells in multiple human organs. Cell Stem Cell 2008;3(3):301–13.
4. De Schauwer C, Meyer E, Van de Walle GR, et al. Markers of stemness in equine mesenchymal stem cells: a plea for uniformity. Theriogenology 2011;75(8):1431–43.
5. Mosna F, Sensebe L, Krampera M. Human bone marrow and adipose tissue mesenchymal stem cells: a user's guide. Stem Cells Dev 2010;19(10):1449–70.
6. Dominici M, Le Blanc K, Mueller I, et al. Minimal criteria for defining multipotent mesenchymal stromal cells. The International Society for Cellular Therapy position statement. Cytotherapy 2006;8(4):315–7.
7. Smith RK, Korda M, Blunn GW, et al. Isolation and implantation of autologous equine mesenchymal stem cells from bone marrow into the superficial digital flexor tendon as a potential novel treatment. Equine Vet J 2003;35(1):99–102.
8. Jacobs RM, Kociba GJ, Ruoff WW. Monoclonal gammopathy in a horse with defective hemostasis. Vet Pathol 1983;20(5):643–7.
9. Durando MM, Zarucco L, Schaer TP, et al. Pneumopericardium in a horse secondary to sternal bone marrow aspiration. Equine Veterinary Education 2006;18:75–9.
10. Kasashima Y, Ueno T, Tomita A, et al. Optimisation of bone marrow aspiration from the equine sternum for the safe recovery of mesenchymal stem cells. Equine Vet J 2011;43(3):288–94.

11. Toupadakis CA, Wong A, Genetos DC, et al. Comparison of the osteogenic potential of equine mesenchymal stem cells from bone marrow, adipose tissue, umbilical cord blood, and umbilical cord tissue. Am J Vet Res 2010;71(10): 1237–45.

12. Kisiday JD, Kopesky PW, Evans CH, et al. Evaluation of adult equine bone marrow- and adipose-derived progenitor cell chondrogenesis in hydrogel cultures. J Orthop Res 2008;26(3):322–31.

13. Vidal MA, Kilroy GE, Lopez MJ, et al. Characterization of equine adipose tissue-derived stromal cells: adipogenic and osteogenic capacity and comparison with bone marrow-derived mesenchymal stromal cells. Vet Surg 2007;36(7):613–22.

14. Vidal MA, Robinson SO, Lopez MJ, et al. Comparison of chondrogenic potential in equine mesenchymal stromal cells derived from adipose tissue and bone marrow. Vet Surg 2008;37(8):713–24.

15. Braun J, Hack A, Weis-Klemm M, et al. Evaluation of the osteogenic and chondrogenic differentiation capacities of equine adipose tissue-derived mesenchymal stem cells. Am J Vet Res 2010;71(10):1228–36.

16. da Silva Meirelles L, Sand TT, Harman RJ, et al. MSC frequency correlates with blood vessel density in equine adipose tissue. Tissue Eng Part A 2009;15(2): 221–9.

17. Koch TG, Heerkens T, Thomsen PD, et al. Isolation of mesenchymal stem cells from equine umbilical cord blood. BMC Biotechnol 2007;7:26.

18. Bartholomew S, Owens SD, Ferraro GL, et al. Collection of equine cord blood and placental tissues in 40 thoroughbred mares. Equine Vet J 2009;41(8):724–8.

19. Bourzac C, Smith LC, Vincent P, et al. Isolation of equine bone marrow-derived mesenchymal stem cells: a comparison between three protocols. Equine Vet J 2010;42(6):519–27.

20. Arnhold SJ, Goletz I, Klein H, et al. Isolation and characterization of bone marrow-derived equine mesenchymal stem cells. Am J Vet Res 2007;68(10):1095–105.

21. Vidal MA, Kilroy GE, Johnson JR, et al. Cell growth characteristics and differentiation frequency of adherent equine bone marrow-derived mesenchymal stromal cells: adipogenic and osteogenic capacity. Vet Surg 2006;35(7):601–10.

22. Wilke MM, Nydam DV, Nixon AJ. Enhanced early chondrogenesis in articular defects following arthroscopic mesenchymal stem cell implantation in an equine model. J Orthop Res 2007;25(7):913–25.

23. Lennon DP, Caplan AI. Isolation of human marrow-derived mesenchymal stem cells. Exp Hematol 2006;34(11):1604–5.

24. Colleoni S, Bottani E, Tessaro I, et al. Isolation, growth and differentiation of equine mesenchymal stem cells: effect of donor, source, amount of tissue and supplementation with basic fibroblast growth factor. Vet Res Commun 2009; 33(8):811–21.

25. Hoynowski SM, Fry MM, Gardner BM, et al. Characterization and differentiation of equine umbilical cord-derived matrix cells. Biochem Biophys Res Commun 2007; 362(2):347–53.

26. Koch TG, Thomsen PD, Betts DH. Improved isolation protocol for equine cord blood-derived mesenchymal stromal cells. Cytotherapy 2009;11(4):443–7.

27. Castro-Malaspina H, Gay RE, Resnick G, et al. Characterization of human bone marrow fibroblast colony-forming cells (CFU-F) and their progeny. Blood 1980; 56(2):289–301.

28. Vidal M, Walker NJ, Napoli E, et al. Evaluation of senescence in mesenchymal stem cells isolated from equine bone marrow, adipose tissue and umbilical cord tissue. Stem Cells Dev May 6, 2011. [Epub ahead of print].

29. Pittenger MF, Mackay AM, Beck SC, et al. Multilineage potential of adult human mesenchymal stem cells. Science 1999;284:143–7.

30. Garvican ER, Vaughan-Thomas A, Redmond C, et al. Chondrocytes harvested from osteochondritis dissecans cartilage are able to undergo limited in vitro chondrogenesis despite having perturbations of cell phenotype in vivo. J Orthop Res 2008;26(8):1133–40.

31. Koerner J, Nesic D, Romero JD, et al. Equine peripheral blood-derived progenitors in comparison to bone marrow-derived mesenchymal stem cells. Stem Cells 2006;24(6):1613–9.

32. Vidal MA, Lopez MJ. Adipogenic differentiation of adult equine mesenchymal stromal cells. Methods Mol Biol 2011;702:61–75.

33. Haack-Sorensen M, Bindslev L, Mortensen S, et al. The influence of freezing and storage on the characteristics and functions of human mesenchymal stromal cells isolated for clinical use. Cytotherapy 2007;9(4):328–37.

34. Mambelli LI, Santos EJ, Frazao PJ, et al. Characterization of equine adipose tissue-derived progenitor cells before and after cryopreservation. Tissue Eng Part C Methods 2009;15(1):87–94.

35. Guest DJ, Smith MR, Allen WR. Monitoring the fate of autologous and allogeneic mesenchymal progenitor cells injected into the superficial digital flexor tendon of horses: preliminary study. Equine Vet J 2008;40(2):178–81.

36. Radcliffe CH, Flaminio MJ, Fortier LA. Temporal analysis of equine bone marrow aspirate during establishment of putative mesenchymal progenitor cell populations. Stem Cells Dev 2010;19(2):269–82.

37. de Mattos Carvalho A, Alves AL, Golim MA, et al. Isolation and immunophenotypic characterization of mesenchymal stem cells derived from equine species adipose tissue. Vet Immunol Immunopathol 2009;132(2–4):303–6.

38. Ibrahim S, Saunders K, Kydd JH, et al. Screening of anti-human leukocyte monoclonal antibodies for reactivity with equine leukocytes. Vet Immunol Immunopathol 2007;119(1–2):63–80.

39. Rozemuller H, Prins HJ, Naaijkens B, et al. Prospective isolation of mesenchymal stem cells from multiple mammalian species using cross-reacting anti-human monoclonal antibodies. Stem Cells Dev 2010;19(12):1911–21.

40. Boucher S, Lakshmipathy U, Vemuri M. A simplified culture and polymerase chain reaction identification assay for quality control performance testing of stem cell media products. Cytotherapy 2009;1–9. [Epub ahead of print].

Autologous Biologic Treatment for Equine Musculoskeletal Injuries: Platelet-Rich Plasma and IL-1 Receptor Antagonist Protein

Jamie Textor, DVM

KEYWORDS

• PRP • Platelet • Horse • IRAP • ACS

We practice equine veterinary medicine in an exciting time: the promise of tissue regeneration and "scarless" healing seems just on the horizon for many types of tissue,[1] and equally within our reach for the unforgiving musculoskeletal tissues of horses. Our clients have access to more information than ever before and are at least as motivated as we are to try new therapies and improve the athletic rehabilitation of their horses. When applied to autologous biologic therapies such as platelet-rich plasma (PRP) and IL-1 receptor antagonist protein (IRAP), this enthusiasm has driven clinical usage to the point that it has outpaced, or perhaps even bypassed, scientific investigation into their use. Unencumbered by the restrictions and testing required for pharmaceuticals, readily available from the patient itself, and with the high safety index of an autologous product, these biologic treatments have been rapidly popularized over the past 5 to 10 years. The concept of an "autograft" is attractive to practitioners and clients alike: the notion of amplifying the patient's own physiology as therapy, to provide a supraphysiologic and perhaps even "regenerative" outcome,

Dr Textor's funding is provided by the UC Davis Center for Equine Health and an NIH Training Grant.

Statement of potential conflict of interest: The author has received 12 PRP and 6 autologous thrombin preparation kits from Harvest Technologies, and 9 E-PET kits from Pall Medical, free of charge, for experimental investigation.

Tablin Laboratory, Department of Pathology, Microbiology and Immunology, College of Veterinary Medicine, University of California Davis, VM3A 4318, 1 Shields Avenue, Davis, CA 95616, USA

E-mail address: jamietextor@gmail.com

Vet Clin Equine 27 (2011) 275–298
doi:10.1016/j.cveq.2011.05.001
0749-0739/11/$ – see front matter © 2011 Elsevier Inc. All rights reserved.

could be considered the ideal treatment. However, the "individualized" or "personalized" nature of these products also makes them difficult to study scientifically or even to draw anecdotal conclusions from—consider that an identical autologous PRP or IRAP product has never been administered to two different patients! The composition of the product, both cellular and soluble, is not only unique for every individual—it is probably often substantially different due to wide interindividual variability. These biologic agents are "cocktail" treatments comprised of many constituent cells and cytokines—in stark contrast to a purified drug preparation containing a single defined, quantified substance with some desired therapeutic action and a milligram-per-kilogram dosage recommendation. In addition, there are multiple preparation systems from which to choose. Further complicating the situation is the fact that these methods have been developed for humans and are generally brought to the veterinary marketplace with little or no validation for equine use. As becomes quickly apparent, there are many variables to consider in the preparation, administration, and composition of biologics such as PRP and IRAP. Although many of these variables are unknown at this time, there is still much to discuss.

Although PRP and IRAP are discussed together in this article, it should be clarified that they are distinct products with wholly different rationales for their use. PRP is used because of the growth-factor content of platelets. Based on the provision of these factors in a highly concentrated form, PRP is intended to support and enhance tissue healing as an anabolic agent. It is probably best used after acute traumatic injury to musculoskeletal tissues. IRAP, on the other hand, has historically been thought of as an anti-catabolic: that is, the predominant goal of its use is to inhibit the inflammatory cascade incited by IL-1, particularly in osteoarthritis (OA), rather than to directly repair or regenerate the tissue. It may be that the prevention of IL-1 activity in and of itself allows for improved endogenous tissue repair, but IRAP has been used most often in the chronic, progressive scenario of OA, rather than for acute injury. Although autologous conditioned serum (ACS) has not historically been considered an anabolic therapy, recent reports have included measurements of its growth factor content.[2,3] Ultimately, the ideal regenerative biologic therapy will likely provide both anabolic and anti-catabolic activities in order to optimize results.[4,5] What PRP and IRAP do have in common is that both are autologous biologic products prepared from whole blood.

This article focuses first on PRP, and then on IRAP, as used for musculoskeletal therapy in horses. Sections are subtitled with the intent that the reader can easily access the information of greatest interest to them, whether that is a review of the nomenclature, the cellular biology behind these therapies, the scientific evidence regarding their use, or simply practical usage information. The article concludes with current questions regarding each product and suggestions for future research to advance our understanding of these biologic agents for musculoskeletal therapy of the horse.

PRP
History and Origin of Use

The concept of platelet-derived therapies arose in the late 1970s to 1980s, as multiple growth factors were discovered within the alpha granules of platelets.[6–8] Initial attempts to augment healing in experimental animal studies used purified single-growth factors, with disappointing results. When platelet lysates were used instead, providing the full complement of growth factors contained within the alpha granules, anabolic effects were observed in a number of wound-healing models. The first clinical use of PRP was reported by Marx in 1998.[9] This seminal study used PRP to supplement cancellous bone graft in the reconstruction of large (>5 cm) mandibular defects in humas. The study was controlled, randomized, blinded, and prospective. In this case, the outcome of interest was bone formation within the defect, and the PRP-treated group demonstrated significant improvements in both radiographic and histologic scores of bone density. Since that time, although the use of PRP to enhance bone formation remains a contentious topic, it has been widely used in oral surgery in humans. Shortly thereafter, multiple reports indicated that PRP produced significant improvements in the healing of complicated wounds in humans.[10] Most recently, PRP has been popularized for use in both human and equine sports medicine, particularly for the treatment of tendon and ligament injuries.[11,12]

PRP Components

Platelets
The therapeutic bases of platelet-derived products derive from the platelet growth factor content and the absolute number of the platelets themselves. Importantly, the contents of alpha granules are only released upon activation of the platelets, and are not constitutively secreted (**Fig. 1**). Platelets contain a potent cargo of over 200 other proteins in their alpha granules, many of which are procoagulant in nature, in addition to the therapeutically desirable growth factors.[13] As hemostatic agents, platelets are designed to secrete these substances only when specifically activated to do so. Adverse effects on the organism resulting from inappropriate granule content release into the bloodstream are thereby prevented. Despite some unsubstantiated comments in the PRP literature,[14,15] there has been no published data to indicate de novo synthesis of growth factors by platelets once they have been fully activated. Platelets do synthesize some proteins upon activation,[16] for up to 2 days after clot formation,[17] but this has not yet been conclusively demonstrated for the growth factors. Current knowledge still maintains that the growth factor content of platelets is produced by the megakaryocyte, and a finite quantity is distributed among the alpha granules of its daughter platelets.[18] Recent data from our laboratory (J.A. Textor, unpublished data, 2011), however, indicates that the sum of platelet-derived growth factor (PDGF) content in an activated equine PRP clot plus the PDGF content in the serum released from that clot is double the amount contained by the same number

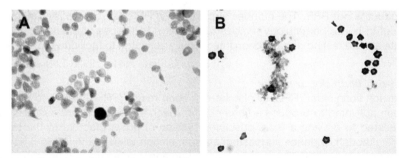

Fig. 1. Cytologic appearance of PRP. Modified Giemsa stain, 100× magnification. (*A*) Resting platelets. With the exception of one erythrocyte, all cells in the field are platelets. Despite the normal variations in platelet shape apparent here, most cells are ovoid in shape and have a smooth outline. The granules can be observed within the platelets. (*B*) Activated platelets with some crenated erythrocytes. The platelets are now almost exclusively found in aggregates, have changed their shape, and are paler in appearance because they have released their granules.

of resting platelets from the same individual. This suggests that new synthesis of growth factors does indeed take place upon activation of the platelets in PRP.

Growth factors
The predominant growth factors in platelets are PDGF and transforming growth factor beta (TGF-β). Vascular endothelial growth factor (VEGF) is known to be present in the platelets of other species and is likely present in equine platelets as well. It is worth noting that TGF-β is released from platelets in its active form.[19] Somewhat surprisingly, growth factor concentrations do not correlate well with platelet number and are highly variable between individuals[20,21] suggesting that other platelet-induced factors may also play a role in platelet-enhanced healing.[22] For more specific information on growth factors the reader is referred to excellent review articles in the literature.[23–25]

Red and white blood cells
The process of concentrating platelets in plasma does not eliminate all other blood cells; leukocytes are also sometimes concentrated by automated preparation systems, and some number of erythrocytes always remains in PRP.

Plasma proteins
As the name suggests, the platelets are concentrated within the plasma fraction of blood, including all of its normal constituent proteins.

Platelet-Derived Products: Definitions

As with many new therapies, the lexicon used to describe platelet-derived products is varied, sometimes confusing, and often redundant. A brief glossary is provided for the reader:

PRP
PRP strictly refers to a plasma product containing platelets at a concentration significantly greater than whole blood. The platelet concentration that defines PRP in humans is $1000 \times 10^3/\mu l$.[14] Equine whole blood platelet counts are slightly lower than typical human counts, but this target concentration seems as reasonable for equine PRP as for the human product. This value was somewhat arbitrarily established, but was based on in vitro studies that showed a dose-dependent treatment response to platelet number.[22,26] If the platelets are not significantly concentrated, the product is not PRP. The number of platelets in PRP can be readily determined by use of in-house hematology analyzers. The term PRP does not indicate whether the platelets are resting or have been intentionally activated to facilitate growth factor release.

Platelet-rich fibrin clot or matrix
Platelet-rich fibrin clot (PRFC) or platelet-rich fibrin matrix (PRFM) refers to PRP that has been activated to produce a fibrin clot, in which the platelets are suspended. It is postulated to provide a more sustained release of growth factors to the treated site,[15,27] although evidence suggests that most elution takes place within 6 hours.[28] As the name implies, PRFC is a solid formulation and its material and handling properties facilitate placement within a surgical wound bed. Depending on the activation method used to generate the fibrin clot—that is, calcium chloride ($CaCl_2$) alone vs thrombin—the growth factor content is likely to vary. PRFC is usually described as being produced by simply recalcifying the anticoagulated PRP by adding 10% $CaCl_2$. Based on the type and concentration of activator, different consistencies of fibrin clot may result; it is also sometimes referred to as a "platelet gel."

Platelet-rich clot releasate

Platelet-rich clot releasate (PRCR) is less frequently encountered in the literature but refers to the supernatant formed once a PRFC contracts. In other words, a PRCR is simply the serum that has been derived from clotting a concentrated number of platelets and, therefore, contains a higher concentration of growth factors than plain serum.

Platelet concentrate

Platelet concentrate (PC) is largely confined to the experimental literature, but refers to a highly concentrated platelet product, well above that conventionally achieved with PRP. In PCs, platelets are suspended in as small a plasma volume as possible.

Current Musculoskeletal Indications for PRP

In horses, PRP is most often used as a percutaneous, ultrasound-guided, intra-lesional treatment for tendon and ligament injuries. It is most often applied as a single injection, but is administered repeatedly per lesion by some clinicians; optimal administration protocols have not been determined. PRP is generally administered as a single agent but alternatively can be applied in combination with stem cells. PRP use for treatment of equine joints has been anecdotally reported,[29,30] although there is currently much less scientific support for treatment of arthropathies than for tendon injuries. In arthroscopic treatment of articular injuries, however, a PRFC can be allowed to set in a chondral defect or injected into a damaged ligament, creating the provisional matrix that is typically absent in the healing of articular tissues.[31] Use of PRP in conjunction with biosynthetic scaffolds also appears promising for osteochondral repair.[32,33]

In humans, successful PRP use has been described for intralesional treatment or augmented surgical reconstruction[34] of acute tendon, ligament, and muscle injuries. PRP is also used for Achilles and patellar tendinopathies, lateral epicondylitis (tennis elbow), plantar fasciitis, and intra-articular applications.[15,35] PRP has been successfully applied during total joint arthroplasty in people and resulted in reduced postoperative pain and earlier hospital discharge compared with controls not receiving PRP[36,37] (these effects were not reproduced for total knee replacement in subsequent studies).[38] These analgesic effects are believed to be related to enhanced hemostasis in cases of total arthroplasty, but anecdotal reports and scientific evidence suggest that primary analgesic effects of PRP may also exist. Stimulation of one of the thrombin receptors (PAR-1) has been shown to increase the pain threshold in laboratory animals via opioid pathways.[39] Thrombin is contained by and released from activated platelets in a positive feedback cycle, such that when activated PRP is administered, thrombin receptors throughout the area are also stimulated and could potentially induce an analgesic response.

Before proceeding to a review of the scientific evidence for PRP, it should be noted that the assessment of PRP's efficacy is fraught by an almost total inconsistency in PRP preparation and administration between studies, in both the human and veterinary fields. The most significant source of variation relates to whether the PRP is used in resting or activated form and, if activated, the method of activation. As mentioned previously, growth factor release by granule secretion does not occur unless platelet activation occurs, by either exogenous or endogenous stimuli. Platelet concentration can also vary widely between preparation systems. These issues are discussed below.

In Vitro Experimental Data

Equine PRP research began with a report on preparation systems by Sutter and colleagues[40] in 2004. The study confirmed that equine platelet concentration and subsequent TGF-β concentration could be achieved using either platelet pheresis or buffy coat methods, which were employed as early platelet concentration methods in humans. A few in vitro studies of PRP effects on equine superficial digital flexor tendon (SDFT) and suspensory ligament explants have been conducted. They demonstrated increased cartilage oligomeric matrix protein production and Type I collagen expression after exposure to PRP, and significantly higher growth factor levels in PRP than in bone marrow preparations.[41–43]

PRP increases in vitro proliferation of a number of cell types, including tenocytes,[44] osteoblasts,[26] and mesenchymal stem cells.[45] PRP treatment of tendon stem cells induces their differentiation into active tenocytes.[46]

PRP growth factor release as induced by variable methods of platelet activation has been only minimally investigated. A study by Martineau and colleagues[47] tested three increasing dosage combinations of thrombin and $CaCl_2$, with the highest dose being that described for clinical human use by Marx in 1998. The investigators found a significant dose-dependent increase in growth factor levels according to activator dose. Activation of equine PRP has been similarly evaluated by the author of this article: the available growth factor content of resting PRP (ie, without exogenous activation) was significantly less than that of plain serum. The concentrations of PDGF-BB and TGF-β were not increased by potential stimuli encountered in the injection process, such as shear or collagen; these factors have previously been postulated to provide "spontaneous" platelet activation upon injection.[48] Subsequent experiments showed that, similar to the Martineau study, a dose-dependent increase in PDGF-BB release was observed with varying doses of bovine thrombin, up to the 143 u/mL concentration used by Marx clinically. Interestingly, when the effect of autologous equine thrombin was compared with matched concentrations of commercially available bovine thrombin (Sigma-Aldrich, St Louis, MO, USA) bovine thrombin induced significant platelet activation as assessed by growth factor release and platelet aggregometry, whereas equine thrombin had little effect on either parameter (J.A. Textor, unpublished data, 2011). Work is underway to investigate this observation.

Experimental Data: In Vivo

PRP treatment in Achilles and patellar tendon healing has been investigated in several studies in rats and rabbits,[49–53] with demonstrable improvement. One set of studies has specifically compared resting versus activated PRP in tendon repair and reported a better outcome with thrombin activation.[51,52] A recent study in dogs addressed the interesting differences in innate repair of intra-articular versus extra-articular ligaments, which is suspected to result from the lack of fibrin clot formation in the former. After treatment with a PRP-collagen hydrogel scaffold, the histologic appearance of experimentally induced cranial cruciate ligament injury sites was significantly better than that of controls. Similarly, injured medial collateral ligaments (MCL) healed better and faster than did the cruciate ligaments; however, after PRP treatment, the histologic quality of cruciate repair matched that of the MCL.[54] PRP appears to enhance neovascularization in healing tissue[55–57] and not only delivers growth factors to the repair site but also induces their endogenous production.[22,58] PRP treatment can enhance the recruitment of presumptive mesenchymal stem cells from the circulation to sites of tendon injury.[53] Evidence to support the use of PRP in osteochondral repair is also increasing.[33,59,60]

A few selected human studies on PRP use for Achilles tendon pathology are presented for comparison here. The de Vos and colleagues[61] study on PRP treatment of degenerative Achilles tendinopathy received notoriety because it was one of few blinded, randomized, placebo-controlled PRP studies in the literature and was published in a prominent journal. In 54 patients, no difference was found between single treatments of saline or resting PRP. These results should be considered along with other details of the study: no information was provided on the PRP in terms of platelet or growth factor content, and the outcome assessment was by patient questionnaire only, with no imaging or quantitative functional indices, as is unfortunately standard for many human studies. Nonetheless, based on available evidence it must be concluded that PRP treatment of chronic tendinopathy is unlikely to be more effective than rehabilitation alone.

Two other human studies on PRP treatment for Achilles rupture did use quantifiable functional outcomes. Sanchez and colleagues[34] reported on a small group of athletes in which surgical reconstruction of the Achilles tendon either was augmented with PRP or was not; all reconstructions were performed by the same surgeon and post-operative rehabilitation was the same between groups. The results were striking: PRP-treated patients had restored range of motion by 7 versus 11 weeks, were running by 11 versus 18 weeks, and had significantly smaller tendon cross-sectional areas (CSA) during weight-bearing (three times the contralateral normal tendon CSA vs five times in controls). However, a more recent study by Schepull and colleagues[62] also evaluated PRP treatment in patients with Achilles rupture, in a larger and more diverse patient population (aged 18–60), with randomized treatment assignment, patients blinded to treatment, and 1-year follow-up. Functional outcomes in this study were indices of tendon elastic modulus, in which no significant differences were detected between groups, and patient questionnaire scores, which were lower in the PRP-treated group ($P<.014$). Interestingly, the platelet count of the PRP was roughly five times higher in this study than the Sanchez report; both were activated with $CaCl_2$ but Sanchez applied the entire prepared PRP fraction, both as a PRFM (clot) overlying the tenorrhaphy site, and also the PRCR by intratendinous injection. In the Schepull study, only the PRCR was used.

In horses, clinical use of PRP was reported for severe mid-body suspensory desmitis in nine Standardbred racehorses.[11] After a controlled rehabilitation program, all horses returned to racing at approximately 8 months after injury and raced for at least 2 years, with an equal number of starts as performed by nine uninjured horses. Despite the lack of true controls and small numbers in this study, the results were impressive: only a single (activated) PRP treatment was performed, the injuries were severe and deemed likely to be career-ending, and post-PRP return to racing occurred in less than 1 year and was sustainable for a normal number of starts thereafter.

Results of PRP treatment in an experimental model of equine SDFT injury has been reported by Bosch and colleagues.[56,63] A single (resting) PRP treatment was performed at 7 days after injury and 6-month endpoints were assessed in comparison to saline-injected control lesions. PRP-treated sites had significantly greater cellularity, collagen and glycosaminoglycan contents, better histologic organization, and more neovascularization than controls. Perhaps most impressively, PRP treatment resulted in stronger tendons: the treated group had increased force-to-failure, which, although modest in degree (about 1.5 times that of controls), was statistically significant.

PRP Preparation

PRP preparation has been conventionally performed by serial centrifugation, initially of whole blood and then the plasma fraction. Platelet-poor plasma is drawn off and the remaining platelet (and leukocyte) sediment is resuspended in a smaller volume of plasma to produce PRP. This can be achieved using standard blood tubes and laboratory centrifuges, with manual transfer between centrifugation steps, or by automated proprietary systems that usually employ a partitioned, disposable collection container and a complementary centrifuge in which it is designed to fit. Although manual preparation is certainly possible, it is more labor-intensive and time-intensive and does require more attention to maintain the sterility of the product.[64] Whole blood is collected in acid-citrate dextrose (ACD) (ie, one part ACD-A to seven-nine parts whole blood), and should be kept warm or at room temperature until centrifugation. In the author's laboratory, preparation of equine PRP is as follows: the whole blood is spun at 200 g for 15 minutes, the plasma is drawn off sterilely and transferred to a new tube, and that plasma is then spun at 400 g for 15 minutes. Platelets will pellet at the bottom of the tube; excess plasma is drawn off and the platelets are gently resuspended with a pipette in whatever residual volume of plasma is desirable for use. Significant platelet concentration can be achieved ($1000 \times 10^3/\mu l$) in most horses using this protocol but, as can occur for any PRP preparation system, it should be noted that individual variation in platelet reactivity occurs. In some horses, premature activation and a lower recovered platelet count can occur, as with any preparation system (**Figs. 2–5**).

There are many commercial PRP centrifuge systems available (SmartPReP2, Harvest Technologies, Plymouth MA, USA; Vet-Stem, Poway, CA, USA; ProTec, Pulse Veterinary Technologies, Alpharetta, GA, USA; Magellan, Arteriocyte Medical Systems, Hopkinton, MA, USA; GPSII Biomet, Biomet Biologics, Inc, Warsaw, IN, USA; Secquire, PPAI Medical, Fort Myers, FL, USA); the systems that have been used successfully in scientific reports of equine PRP are Harvest SmartPReP2,[41–43,48] Secquire,[11,40] and GPSII Biomet.[56,63] Most systems produce 7 mL of PRP from 54 mL of whole blood. The advantages of these systems are ease of use, rapid production of PRP, and maintenance of sterility. Although the direct comparison of multiple commercial PRP systems is beyond the scope of this article and the author's own research thus far, the information provided here should aid practitioners in their evaluation of these systems for equine use. The main considerations are the platelet concentration of the resultant PRP and the avoidance of premature platelet activation (which can cause growth factor release into the whole plasma fraction, and therefore result in lower growth factor concentrations in the treatment syringe). However, for most systems, all literature and data provided by the manufacturer is in reference to human PRP. Species differences exist in platelet size, optimal centrifugation protocol for their isolation, and platelet reactivity, and therefore manufacturers that provide data specific to equine PRP for their systems must be considered preferable to those that cannot. Common sense must also be employed. If, for instance, a system "does not require anticoagulants," then it should be obvious that the system produces only a clot and plain serum, not a platelet-concentrated product.

A different preparation system (E-PET, Pall Animal Health, Port Washington, NY, USA) is available for stall-side PRP preparation by gravity filtration of platelets only. The system is user-friendly and appears to provide significant platelet concentration; PRP is produced in 10 minutes without the need for a centrifuge.

PRP Administration

PRP administration is most often performed by percutaneous intra-lesional injection, using sterile technique and usually under ultrasonographic guidance. Many practitioners use resting PRP without any activation. Although growth factor delivery is likely to be significantly less with the use of resting than activated PRP, the study by Bosch and colleagues[63] demonstrated positive effects by use of resting PRP. It should be noted that in Bosch's study, the reported growth factor concentrations were

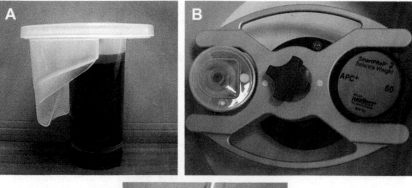

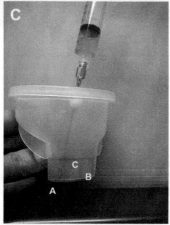

Fig. 2. Methods of PRP Preparation. Automated centrifugation: Harvest SmartPReP2. (*A*) Citrated whole blood has been injected into the main compartment of the disposable container. (*B*) The container is placed in the centrifuge opposite a counterweight, and a preprogrammed centrifugation cycle is performed. (*C*) After centrifugation, the packed red cells are retained in "A," the platelet layer is labeled "B," and the platelet-poor plasma is "C." Excess platelet-poor plasma is being aspirated, and the platelet layer will then be resuspended in the residual volume.

measured after a sample of the PRP had been frozen and thawed (G. Bosch, personal communication, 2010) and do not, therefore, represent the available growth factor concentrations in the lesion site (ie, the PRP used for treatment had not been frozen). This provides a useful segue into current recommendations for PRP activation, as freezing and thawing platelets is an effective, safe, and well-known method of inducing growth factor release.[41,65] Although the freezing process introduces another step and delay in the preparation cycle, it can be expedited by use of liquid nitrogen and rapid thawing in a water bath. Using this protocol, the platelets are partially activated and lysed, causing passive leakage of growth factors from the cells, and the PRP formulation remains liquid. Frozen aliquots can also be banked for future use. The quantity of PDGF-BB released after freezing has been shown to be equivalent to that released after treatment with a low (1 u/mL) dose of bovine thrombin.[65] Alternatively, PRP can simply be recalcified with 10% $CaCl_2$, to a final concentration of 3.4 mg/mL (23 mM)[34] in PRP. For example, to make a total volume of 7 mL, 6.75 mL of PRP is placed in a red top tube and 0.25 mL of 10%$CaCl_2$ is added. The tube is

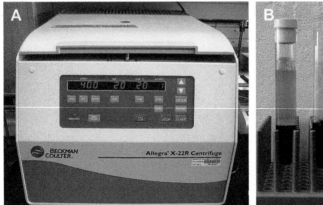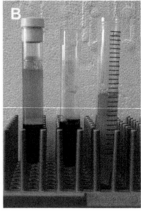

Fig. 3. Methods of PRP Preparation. Standard serial centrifugation. (*A*) Using a standard laboratory centrifuge, tubes of citrated whole blood are spun to separate the plasma and platelets from the erythrocytes. (*B*) The tube on the left has been spun once to separate the plasma and platelets from the erythrocytes; the plasma has been transferred from the middle tube to the tube on the right. Using a second centrifugation cycle, the platelets within that plasma are concentrated into a pellet and then resuspended into a lesser volume.

incubated at 37°C for 30 to 60 minutes, and a platelet-rich fibrin clot will form in the tube. (With more time, more clot retraction will occur and a greater volume of platelet-rich clot releasate is available for injection.) If treatment is to be administered surgically rather than percutaneously, the clot fraction should also be used for maximum growth factor concentration at the site. The growth factor concentrations from $CaCl_2$-activated PRP are higher than those derived from a freeze-thaw cycle (J.A. Textor, unpublished data, 2011).

Xenogeneic thrombin has been safely used in horses. The Waselau and colleagues[11] study used approximately 2 units of bovine thrombin per milliliter of PRP and a wound-healing study reported use of 20 units of human thrombin[66] per milliliter of PRP. When used, thrombin is added during the administration process via a dual syringe, or (depending on concentration) can be mixed into the PRP directly and either injected immediately or used as a platelet-rich fibrin clot. Until recently, all human-activated PRP use had employed 10% $CaCl_2$ and purified bovine thrombin, at a supraphysiologic concentration,[14] with very few adverse effects reported. Although $CaCl_2$ is often used in combination with thrombin, it is not necessary. Platelets contain enough intracellular calcium to proceed with the activation cascade even in an anti-coagulated sample.[67] Nonetheless, thrombin is not a benign protein. Although it continues to cause dose-dependent growth factor release even well above physiologic levels, adverse effects in cell and tissue culture models have been observed in association with high thrombin concentrations.[68] Until further studies are completed, recommendations for methods of thrombin use cannot yet be stated for horses. $CaCl_2$ can be used alone as an activator of PRP, although it is slower and less potent than is thrombin. The conceptual advantages to platelet activation during the administration of PRP, rather than simply platelet lysis as induced by freezing, are (1) greater growth factor release is induced by the active, cytoskeletally-driven process of granule secretion and (2) the resulting clot serves as a provisional matrix within the wound bed, serving as a scaffold, which should enhance tissue repair.

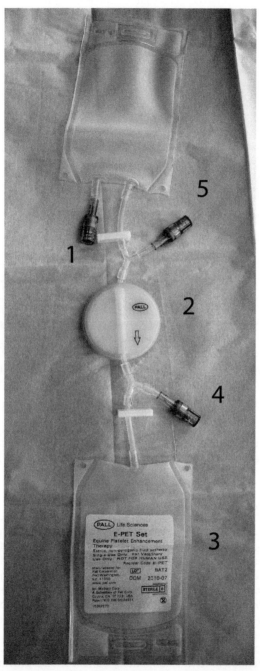

Fig. 4. Methods of PRP Preparation. Gravity filtration: Pall Equine Platelet Enhancement Therapy ("E-PET"). This system does not require centrifugation. Citrated whole blood is injected via a port (1), then flows by gravity through a filter (2) that retains the majority of platelets and some leukocytes. The majority of the plasma and the erythrocytes pass through the filter into the waste bag (3). The platelets are then back-flushed out of the filter by injecting 2% sodium chloride at a second port (4) and collecting the platelet-rich product in a syringe attached to a third port (5).

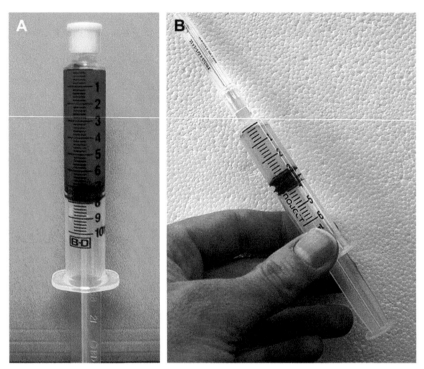

Fig. 5. Different preparations yield different PRP products. The color of PRP varies depending on the number of contaminating erythrocytes, and can range from blood-tinged (A) to straw-colored (B) in appearance.

Costs

Disposable collection containers are usually about $250 each; centrifuge prices vary widely in the range of $2000 to $4000. Client costs for a single PRP treatment are usually in the range of $600 to $1000.

Safety

As an autologous biologic product, PRP is considered an extremely safe therapeutic agent. However, it should be borne in mind that platelets are also inflammatory cells, and that leukocytes are also present in PRP. Acute pain after injection is sometimes reported in humans and horses. Patient observation is recommended for at least 15 minutes after PRP administration; if pain or swelling is observed at the site of injection, icing the limb is recommended. Although nonsteroidal use is avoided in human medicine because of the significant platelet inhibition that results and concerns about thereby reducing PRP treatment efficacy, this concern is unfounded if the platelets have been delivered in an already activated state. In any case, equine platelets show little inhibition in response to phenylbutazone or naproxen.[69] Therefore, the use of these substances for anti-inflammatory benefit should provide no interference with PRP treatment.

CURRENT QUESTIONS: DIRECTIONS FOR FUTURE RESEARCH

"A review of the literature reveals a rampant lack of standardization in the preparation of PRP; consequently, it is problematic when attempting to extrapolate data

from 1 study to the next. The lack of standardized protocol to produce and eval-uate PRP in the literature can help explain the inconsistent clinical and experi-mental results."

—Foster, 2009.[15]

In the author's opinion, these are the most pressing questions pertaining to musculo-skeletal use of PRP in horses as well as in other species:

1. By what metric should PRP quality be assessed? Is it platelet number, growth factor concentration, or something else that is most strongly correlated with ther-apeutic effect?
2. Is one preparation method superior to another for production of equine PRP? Is there a difference in therapeutic outcome whether PRP is applied in a resting or activated state? What is the optimal protocol for PRP preparation and administra-tion in horses?
3. Does PRP work to aid repair in other musculoskeletal injuries, such as fractures, muscle tears, or articular lesions? Does it really work for acute tendon and ligament injuries in horses? Although there is currently evidence to suggest that it does, there is not much of it. More studies of both experimental injury models as well as controlled clinical trials of PRP use are required to further substantiate its use as a valid musculoskeletal therapy in horses.
4. There is a need to define the basic, and then the tissue and site-specific, factors that optimize tissue repair, which can eventually be harnessed to truly regenerate it. Marked variability in healing occurs even within the same tissue type at different anatomic locations.[54,70] This issue is obviously more than just a question in a list; rather, it is this type of information that will truly serve as the foundation for regen-erative medicine. Until we know what the target is, in terms of the ideal type and composition of regenerative therapy for a given anatomic site, we are simply proceeding by trial and error.

SUMMARY: PRP

Scientific evidence indicates that PRP can provide a scaffold and growth factor concentrate to enhance the cellular repair of musculoskeletal lesions. PRP is an attractive product because of its autologous nature, noninvasive collection process, and rapid preparation. If disposables and equipment costs are minimized, there is no reason that PRP should not also be an affordable product for clients. Buyers should beware of the various "PRP" preparation systems in the marketplace—as practi-tioners we have a responsibility to ensure that what we are selling our clients as "PRP" actually is platelet-rich plasma. Once prepared, platelet activation of PRP is important to maximize growth factor release. Work is underway to optimize PRP administration protocols for the horse.

IRAP OR ACS
History and Origin of Use

In 1986, identification of an endogenous IRAP was reported by Balavoine and colleagues,[71] who had serendipitously discovered the substance in the urine of three febrile, leukemic patients. Its anti-IL-1 properties were demonstrated by its ability to decrease collagenase and prostaglandin (PGE_2) production induced by IL-1 in cultured fibroblasts, and it was determined that the cellular source of this antagonist was the monocyte or macrophage. Investigators next determined that its production could be induced by culturing normal monocytes on surfaces that activated them. This occurred simultaneously with the production of IL-1 itself, suggesting a regulatory function for this peptide in normal physiology. In 1990, Hannum and colleagues[72] reported that the specific mechanism of IL-1 antagonism was taking place at the IL-1 receptor itself, and that the inhibitory peptide was a pure, specific antagonist with no agonist activity. Although other endogenous functional IL-1 antagonists also exist,[73] it was this 17 kDa specific receptor antagonist that became known as "IL-1 ra" or "IRAP." Given that IL-1 was considered the "master cytokine" in so many diseases, not least of all in inflammatory arthropathies, the therapeutic potential of this substance induced huge excitement across medicine and, in 1997, the equine IRAP gene was cloned at the University of Tokyo.[74] Since that time, there have been several well-designed experimental studies that support the use of IRAP in horses, by intra-articular administration of either ACS or the IRAP gene itself.[4,75–77]

Musculoskeletal Indications for ACS Use as Currently Practiced

In horses, ACS has most often been used for intra-articular treatment of OA. It is also used by some surgeons prophylactically, for its anti-inflammatory and chondroprotective effects following arthroscopy. There is support for this practice experimentally, in that most in vivo IRAP studies have employed models of early OA, such as chip fracture[75,76] or cruciate ligament transection,[78] and have demonstrated positive responses to IRAP therapy.

In human medicine, IRAP is used for intra-articular treatment of rheumatoid arthritis[79] and ACS is used for OA, for lumbar pain of neurogenic origin (by perineural injection), and for muscle injury (by direct intralesional injection).[2] Recently, a 6-hour incubation period has been described in human medicine but, since IRAP production is known to be linear over time for up to 36 hours,[2] the 6-hour ACS contains substantially less IRAP than ACS incubated for 24 hours.[80]

Composition and Nomenclature

> "…the exact composition of this souplike mixture is still unknown…"
> —Frisbie, 2007.[76]

Although commonly referred to it as "IRAP" in equine practice, the product is more correctly called ACS. In 2003, founders of the German company, Orthokine, reported on their variation of IRAP production by physicochemical methods.[81] They had developed a syringe system containing glass beads, by which practitioners could perform a 24-hour blood culture and then collect an IRAP-enhanced serum product. However, as the quote above aptly indicates, ACS is actually an acellular composite of many blood-derived substances, not a purified protein as the term "IRAP" suggests, and this uncertainty may have a number of as-yet-undetermined implications. In this respect, more attention has recently been paid to the other cytokine constituents of ACS, such as the pro-inflammatory cytokines IL-1 itself, TNF-α, and IL-6, the anti-inflammatory IL-10, and growth factors.[2,3,81]

The term "cytokine" refers to a small soluble protein that has pleiotropic effects on target cells, whether in an autocrine, paracrine, or endocrine manner. The term describes both pro-inflammatory and anti-inflammatory substances and activities, and "growth factors" are considered to be cytokines. The growth factor content of ACS has been sporadically quantified: based on data from at least 80 human subjects from whom ACS was prepared by 6-hour incubation, TGF-β concentrations in ACS were 98 times that of whole blood, and PDGF-AB and VEGF were 19 and 8 times the whole blood content, respectively.[2] It should be borne in mind that any serum product contains significantly more growth factors than whole blood, as they are released from platelets during the clotting cascade. Of the growth factors, TGF-β and IGF-1 are considered to be chondroprotectants; TGF-β also downregulates IL-1. In the only report of growth factor content in equine ACS, IGF-1 levels were double that of plain serum and TGF-β levels were no different from serum concentrations.[3]

In Vitro Experimental Data

Equine IRAP is 21 kDa and comprised of 177 amino acids, with 76% homology to the human protein.[70] IRAP is produced predominantly by monocytes and, to a much lesser extent, by keratinocytes and neutrophils; the production of IRAP takes place simultaneously with IL-1 production by the same cell.[82] IRAP production can be induced by a number of means in the laboratory, including exposure to surface-bound IgG, LPS, IL-1 itself, or even medical grade glass surfaces devoid of any agonist,[2,81,82] as it is produced for clinical use. By virtue of its specific receptor antagonism, IRAP blocks IL-1 activity in all conventional experimental assays (collagenase and PGE_2 production, fibroblast proliferation, and T cell proliferation).[71–73,83] Blockade of articular IL-1 effects by IRAP prevents the cartilage matrix breakdown induced by matrix metalloproteinases and helps restore proteoglycan and Type II collagen production.[4,84]

However, because IL-1 is such a potent cytokine, the ratio of IRAP to IL-1 must be quite high to prevent IL-1's effects. Each fibroblast has literally thousands of IL-1 receptors on its surface,[85] and yet cellular responses to IL-1 are induced by the binding of only a few receptors. Since the binding affinities of IRAP and IL-1 to the IL-1 receptor are considered equivalent, effective antagonism of IL-1 requires that the available IL-1 peptides must be significantly outnumbered by IRAP peptides. Therefore, the ratio of IRAP to IL-1 in synovial fluid after treatment is considered to be more useful index of efficacy than the absolute concentrations of each protein, and the necessary ratio for 50% inhibition of IL-1 activity has been determined to be roughly 100:1 for human chondrocytes, and 30:1 for human synoviocytes.[73] The administration of 2 mL ACS to a human osteoarthritic knee has been calculated to provide an IRAP/IL-1 ratio of 170:1, based on the typical IL-1 concentration of human osteoarthritic synovial fluid.[81] The therapeutically desirable ratio in horses has not been specifically determined.

Although previous reports indicated there was no attendant increase in IL-1 itself or TNF-α in ACS, more recent studies in both human and equine ACS confirm that these undesirable cytokines are increased in ACS, in conjunction with the increase in IRAP.[80] In the equine study,[3] IL-1 β was increased four-fold in both ACS and 24-hour serum. IRAP itself was also elevated (82-fold) in plain serum after a 24-hour incubation period, without any special manipulation of the sample, and this concentration was not significantly different from that of the ACS. This recent work has called the ACS product into some question and suggests that the composition of ACS, at least for those constituents that have been measured by investigators, may not be effectively different from 24-hour-old serum. The investigators concluded that the positive results previously ascribed to IRAP activity may instead be due to other undetermined factors within the ACS.

In Vivo Experimental Data

Laboratory animal studies

IRAP has been shown to reduce morbidity in a diverse range of animal disease models, including endotoxemia, inflammatory bowel disease, and OA. One early example of the significant chondroprotection of IRAP was reported by Caron and colleagues[78] in 1996, using a cruciate transection OA model in dogs. Intra-articular injection of recombinant human IRAP was performed twice weekly for 4 weeks, beginning at the time of surgery, and was compared with a control group treated with saline injections. At the 4-week endpoint of the study, there was a significant dose-dependent improvement in gross and histologic scores as well as number of cartilage lesions in the IRAP-treated group. IRAP could be detected in the synovial fluid of all treated animals, whereas it was not detected in the synovial fluid of controls, suggesting that endogenous intra-articular production of the substance was relatively low. It is important to note that this study used the recombinant IRAP peptide, not ACS. The reader is referred to existing review articles for the many other citations of studies using laboratory animals.[5,86] When considering the results of these studies, it should be borne in mind that experimental models of OA are very early representations of the disease process, with intervention often provided at the time of or shortly after insult. Not surprisingly, the same results are more difficult to obtain in naturally occurring, chronic clinical disease.

Human studies

Recombinant IRAP has become standard-of-care therapy for rheumatoid arthritis in people[87] but unfortunately, despite favorable results in experimental animal models of OA, the results of large clinical trials of either recombinant IRAP or ACS treatment for OA in people have been disappointing overall.[79,88–91] One large multicenter prospective trial in Germany was reported in 2009,[92] in which 376 patients with knee OA were divided into three groups and received intra-articular injections of ACS, hyaluronic acid, or saline, with both the patients and the examiners blinded to treatment. All groups demonstrated improvement from baseline, with the ACS group demonstrating significantly greater improvement than the other groups. Unfortunately, both "control" groups in this study received only three injections, whereas the ACS group received six injections, thereby invalidating the notion of a control and seriously weakening the results of the study. Some prominent investigators have suggested that the recombinant IRAP product used in rheumatoid arthritis, anakinra, may indeed prove useful for OA as a repeated dosing strategy, rather than the single-dose approach employed in the Chevalier and colleagues[79] study. Others suggest that, because of the apparently short half-life of the peptide itself in humans, gene therapy is a better approach to deliver the IL-1 antagonist, to induce sustained in situ production of the protein. Interestingly, in both dogs and horses, the synovial fluid half-life of either the human recombinant IRAP or IRAP from ACS appears to be of longer duration[76,78] than has been reported in people.[79]

Horse studies

Equine surgeon-scientists have made significant contributions to the study of IRAP and its genetic delivery in particular.[4,75,77,93] In fact, intra-articular delivery of IRAP by gene therapy[75] actually preceded the use of ACS[76] in the horse. Transduction of synovial fibroblasts by an adenoviral vector carrying the IRAP gene was first performed in vitro, with consequent IRAP production by the transduced cells in culture. The IRAP vector was next introduced into the normal carpi of experimental horses to determine the correct viral dose and newly produced IRAP concentrations were detected in the synovial fluid for up to 28 days. Finally, the IRAP vector was delivered to horses with early OA, induced by the Colorado State University carpal chip model, 14 days after the initial insult. Significant adverse effects of treatment were not detected; although, unsurprisingly, the leukocyte count was higher in joints treated with the viral vector. Improvements in lameness, synovial effusion, gross lesions, and cartilage proteoglycan preservation were reported for the treated group. In the

ACS study,[76] the chip model was again employed and intra-articular injections of ACS were performed weekly for 4 weeks, beginning 2 weeks after surgery, and compared with saline-injected controls. As is standard for this model, the horses were also exercised 5 days per week during the study, a more critical test than the common clinical practice of reducing activity after ACS administration. Lameness was significantly improved in the ACS-treated group at 70 days after injury (grade 1/5 vs 2/5 in saline-treated horses) and, interestingly, IRAP was still detectable in the synovial fluid at this time, despite being 35 days after the last ACS treatment. Despite the clinical improvement, no improvements in histologic or gross lesions were detected, and the investigators concluded that IRAP delivery by gene therapy had produced a better outcome than that obtained by ACS treatment. To date, this is the only published scientific report of ACS treatment for OA in horses.

Another gene therapy study was reported by Morisset and colleagues[77] in 2007, in which full thickness cartilage defects were created in the stifle and carpus. Horses were treated with an adenoviral vector carrying IRAP and IGF-1 at the time of surgery. In this study, no significant differences were seen between treated animals and controls. IRAP levels in synovial fluid were detected for 3 weeks after vector transfection.

Anecdotal Comments

Although, as a profession, we should be diligent in producing and reviewing scientific data to inform our clinical choices, as practitioners we ultimately practice according to our own experience and the respected opinions of our colleagues. For this reason and until data on clinical use of ACS in horses becomes available, a brief synopsis of anecdotal reports is presented here based on informal personal communications. Overall, the product appears to be favorably viewed and endorsed by practitioners with a large, athletic patient base, which should provide a critical population needed to assess its efficacy. ACS seems particularly popular with sport horse practitioners and, in particular, when positive drug tests for pharmaceuticals need to be avoided during the active show season. Many practitioners report that ACS "works when steroids stop working," and apply it to more chronic cases that have been undergoing regular intraarticular treatment to maintain an osteoarthritic joint. In the Orthokine product literature (Düsseldorf, Germany), Thomas Weinberger of the Equine Burg Clinic Müggenhausen writes that ACS use in horses of mixed disciplines resulted in resolution of lameness for at least 3 months in 178 out of 262 horses. The client cost for ACS appears to limit its use; many practitioners indicate that they would use ACS more often if their clients could afford it. Improvement in lameness is generally expected after the second but not first injection, with resolution of lameness after the third or fourth injection. Duration of effect has been reported to vary from 3 months to 1 year, when used for joints that had been unresponsive or only briefly responsive to other intra-articular therapies. There is some debate about whether combination therapy using corticosteroids and/or prophylactic antibiotics is indicated; most practitioners appear to use ACS alone. Adverse effects are reported to occur rarely, as for biologics in general.

The successful use of ACS for intra-lesional treatment of suspensory desmitis and flexor tendinitis is also described by some practitioners; the author is aware that studies are underway to investigate the in vitro effects of IRAP products on tenocytes.

Preparation and Administration

ACS is produced by aseptic collection of approximately 50 mL of whole blood into a 60 mL proprietary syringe or container, which is filled with approximately 200 small beads made of medical-grade borosilicate glass. The beads have a surface area of roughly 21 mm^2 and are 2.5 mm in diameter; the interaction of monocytes with the bead surfaces is believed to lead to IRAP production.[81] After an incubation period of 24 hours at 37°C, the syringe is spun in a compatible proprietary centrifuge at 2500 to 3100 g for 10 minutes, and the resulting autologous conditioned serum is aspirated. Filtered aliquots of 2 mL are usually prepared, and those not used for immediate treatment are frozen at −20°C for future use. To prevent proteolytic degradation of the therapeutic peptides in ACS, it should be refrigerated until use, consistent with general good laboratory practice. IRAP administration is performed using sterile technique, and usually employs a 2 mL injection once per week for 4 weeks.

There are currently two manufacturers of ACS for equine use and the resultant ACS from each has recently been compared.[3] The German company, Orthogen, originally developed and marketed the preparation system named Orthokine for human use. The system is available in the United States under the trade name "irap," supplied by Dechra Veterinary Products. The other manufacturer is Arthrex, which produces the "IRAPII" system. Based on the results of the study by Hraha and colleagues,[3] the IRAP content was significantly higher in the Arthrex ACS than in the Orthogen ACS, although the former product also contained more IL-1β. Ultimately the ratios of IRAP to IL-1 content in the ACS were not significantly different between products, but the IRAPII ACS was the only product to show a ratio that was significantly higher than that in baseline serum. There was no significant difference in IL-10, IL-1 β, TNF-α, IGF-1, or TGF-β content of the two ACS products. The IRAP content in the Arthrex product was significantly greater than that of the Orthogen product; the Orthogen IRAP concentration was no different from that of plain serum after 24-hour incubation. These results were in contrast to results reported for human blood, and the investigators emphasize the point mentioned in the introduction of this article: autologous biologic preparation devices marketed for horses should be evaluated specifically for use in the horse, rather than based on human data.

Costs

Current pricing for ACS centrifuge and rotor systems is approximately $5500 from each manufacturer. Preparation kits cost approximately $250 each and each kit yields roughly 10 mL of ACS. Depending on the volume of ACS prepared and including charges for time, labor, and expertise, client costs at most hospitals usually exceed $1000 to $1500 for a course of four ACS treatments.

Current Questions on ACS Use for Musculoskeletal Treatment in Horses

Does it work (ie, reduce clinical signs) in horses with naturally occurring OA?
Although there is anecdotal support for the efficacy of ACS, only one controlled experimental study has been performed to investigate its efficacy.[76] The study used a well-established, induced model of early OA and demonstrated statistically significant positive outcomes in clinical variables, supporting the use of the product. The improvements were mild to moderate and were detected in comparison to a saline, not serum, placebo control. Results after gene delivery of IRAP in the same model were deemed better than those attained in the ACS study. As is true for PRP, to truly evaluate the efficacy of ACS, our field needs at least one large clinical study with matched, true control subjects and blinded evaluators.

If it does work, which components are responsible for the therapeutic result?
This is a challenging question to answer. It requires comprehensive compositional analysis of a large number of ACS samples, perhaps by multiplex bead cytokine analysis. The modifications induced by the ACS preparation protocol would need to be

determined, in comparison to plain serum incubated for an equal amount of time, as well as the compositional variability between patients. Associations between ACS composition and outcome after treatment in OA-affected horses could help identify the most important therapeutic component or components; whether it is the absolute IRAP content or a particular "recipe" of several factors that results in superior therapeutic results. For this latter assessment, all subjects would need to have the same insult (ie, an experimental OA model) to facilitate comparison.

Although recent studies have suggested that other constituent cytokines of ACS besides IRAP may also be of therapeutic importance,[2,3,80,90] it should be restated that there is huge body of experimental evidence, derived from a range of in vitro and in vivo models, indicating that IL-1 is central in the pathogenesis of OA,[80,93,94] and that prevention of its action by any of several mechanisms results in attenuation of the disease.[86,94] Whereas a more comprehensive understanding of ACS components is perhaps warranted, we should not forget the expansive evidence supporting IL-1 antagonism as a therapeutic strategy.

SUMMARY: IRAP/ACS

IRAP therapies are considered structure-and disease-modifying OA drugs in concept and theory. In both human and equine OA, therapeutic approaches that target the specific pathophysiologic events of OA are more likely to slow, stop, or even prevent OA, as opposed to the largely palliative actions of conventional mainstay therapy (nonsteroidal anti-inflammatory drugs). Despite promising in vitro and experimental in vivo results of IRAP use, ACS has not proven superior to placebo for the treatment of OA in humans, based on the results of several large, randomized clinical trials. In the field of equine veterinary medicine, however, anecdotal and limited experimental evidence currently supports the use of autologous conditioned serum to treat OA in horses.

REFERENCES

1. Ferguson MW, O'Kane S. Scar-free healing: from embryonic mechanisms to adult therapeutic intervention. Philos Trans R Soc Lond B Biol Sci 2004;359(1445): 839–50.
2. Wehling P, Moser C, Frisbie D, et al. Autologous conditioned serum in the treatment of orthopedic diseases: the orthokine therapy. BioDrugs 2007;21(5):323–32.
3. Hraha TH, Cowley KM, McIlwraith CW, et al. Autologous conditioned serum: the comparative cytokine profiles of two commercial methods (IRAP and IRAP II) using equine blood. Equine Vet J 2011. DOI: 10.1111/j.2042-3306.2010.00321.x.
4. Nixon AJ, Haupt JL, Frisbie DD, et al. Gene-mediated restoration of cartilage matrix by combination insulin-like growth factor-I/interleukin-1 receptor antagonist therapy. Gene Ther 2005;12(2):177–86.
5. Blom AB, van der Kraan PM, van den Berg WB. Cytokine targeting in osteoarthritis. Curr Drug Targets 2007;8(2):283–92.
6. Kaplan DR, Chao FC, Stiles CD, et al. Platelet alpha granules contain a growth factor for fibroblasts. Blood 1979;53(6):1043–52.
7. Assoian RK, Komoriya A, Meyers CA, et al. Transforming growth factor-beta in human platelets. Identification of a major storage site, purification, and characterization. J Biol Chem 1983;258(11):7155–60.
8. Karey KP, Sirbasku DA. Human platelet-derived mitogens. II. Subcellular localization of insulinlike growth factor I to the alpha-granule and release in response to thrombin. Blood 1989;74(3):1093–100.

9. Marx RE, Carlson ER, Eichstaedt RM, et al. Platelet-rich plasma: growth factor enhancement for bone grafts. Oral Surg Oral Med Oral Pathol Oral Radiol Endod 1998;85(6):638–46.

10. Mazzucco L, Medici D, Serra M, et al. The use of autologous platelet gel to treat difficult-to-heal wounds: a pilot study. Transfusion 2004;44(7):1013–8.

11. Waselau M, Sutter WW, Genovese RL, et al. Intralesional injection of platelet-rich plasma followed by controlled exercise for treatment of midbody suspensory ligament desmitis in Standardbred racehorses. J Am Vet Med Assoc 2008;232(10): 1515–20.

12. Sampson S, Gerhardt M, Mandelbaum B. Platelet rich plasma injection grafts for musculoskeletal injuries: a review. Curr Rev Musculoskelet Med 2008;1(3–4): 165–74.

13. Blair P, Flaumenhaft R. Platelet alpha-granules: basic biology and clinical correlates. Blood Rev 2009;23(4):177–89.

14. Marx RE. Platelet-rich plasma: evidence to support its use. J Oral Maxillofac Surg 2004;62(4):489–96.

15. Foster TE, Puskas BL, Mandelbaum BR, et al. Platelet-rich plasma: from basic science to clinical applications. Am J Sports Med 2009;37(11):2259–72.

16. Zimmerman GA, Weyrich AS. Signal-dependent protein synthesis by activated platelets: new pathways to altered phenotype and function. Arterioscler Thromb Vasc Biol 2008;28(3):s17–24.

17. Weyrich AS, Dixon DA, Pabla R, et al. Signal-dependent translation of a regulatory protein, Bcl-3, in activated human platelets. Proc Natl Acad Sci U S A 1998; 95(10):5556–61.

18. Antoniades HN. PDGF: a multifunctional growth factor. Baillieres Clin Endocrinol Metab 1991;5(4):595–613.

19. Blakytny R, Ludlow A, Martin GE, et al. Latent TGF-beta1 activation by platelets. J Cell Physiol 2004;199(1):67–76.

20. Roussy Y, Bertrand Duchesne MP, Gagnon G. Activation of human platelet-rich plasmas: effect on growth factors release, cell division and in vivo bone formation. Clin Oral Implants Res 2007;18(5):639–48.

21. Weibrich G, Kleis WK, Kunz-Kostomanolakis M, et al. Correlation of platelet concentration in platelet-rich plasma to the extraction method, age, sex, and platelet count of the donor. Int J Oral Maxillofac Implants 2001;16(5): 693–9.

22. Giacco F, Perruolo G, D'Agostino E, et al. Thrombin-activated platelets induce proliferation of human skin fibroblasts by stimulating autocrine production of insulin-like growth factor-1. FASEB J 2006;20(13):2402–4.

23. Molloy T, Wang Y, Murrell G. The roles of growth factors in tendon and ligament healing. Sports Med 2003;33(5):381–94.

24. Zachos TA, Bertone AL. Growth factors and their potential therapeutic applications for healing of musculoskeletal and other connective tissues. Am J Vet Res 2005;66(4):727–38.

25. Barrientos S, Stojadinovic O, Golinko MS, et al. Growth factors and cytokines in wound healing. Wound Repair Regen 2008;16(5):585–601.

26. Ogino Y, Ayukawa Y, Kukita T, et al. The contribution of platelet-derived growth factor, transforming growth factor-beta1, and insulin-like growth factor-I in platelet-rich plasma to the proliferation of osteoblast-like cells. Oral Surg Oral Med Oral Pathol Oral Radiol Endod 2006;101(6):724–9.

27. Dohan Ehrenfest DM, de Peppo GM, Doglioli P, et al. Slow release of growth factors and thrombospondin-1 in Choukroun's platelet-rich fibrin (PRF): a gold

standard to achieve for all surgical platelet concentrates technologies. Growth Factors 2009;27(1):63–9.

28. Su CY, Kuo YP, Nieh HL, et al. Quantitative assessment of the kinetics of growth factors release from platelet gel. Transfusion 2008;48(11):2414–20.

29. Abellenat I, Prades M. Intraarticular platelet rich plasma (PRP) therapy: evaluation in 42 sport horses with OA. Proceedings of the 11th International Congress of the World Equine Veterinary Association. Guaruja (Brazil); 2009.

30. Fortier L. Current Concepts in Joint Therapy. Proceedings of the 11th International Congress of the World Equine Veterinary Association. Guaruja (Brazil); 2009.

31. Fallouh L, Nakagawa K, Sasho T, et al. Effects of autologous platelet-rich plasma on cell viability and collagen synthesis in injured human anterior cruciate ligament. J Bone Joint Surg Am 2010;92(18):2909–16.

32. Getgood A, Henson F, Brooks R, et al. Platelet-rich plasma activation in combination with biphasic osteochondral scaffolds-conditions for maximal growth factor production. Knee Surg Sports Traumatol Arthrosc 2011. DOI: 10.1007/s00167-011-1456-6.

33. Sun Y, Feng Y, Zhang CQ, et al. The regenerative effect of platelet-rich plasma on healing in large osteochondral defects. Int Orthop 2010;34(4):589–97.

34. Sanchez M, Anitua E, Azofra J, et al. Comparison of surgically repaired Achilles tendon tears using platelet-rich fibrin matrices. Am J Sports Med 2007;35(2):245–51.

35. Filardo G, Kon E, Buda R, et al. Platelet-rich plasma intra-articular knee injections for the treatment of degenerative cartilage lesions and osteoarthritis. Knee Surg Sports Traumatol Arthrosc 2011;19(4):528–35.

36. Gardner MJ, Demetrakopoulos D, Klepchick PR, et al. The efficacy of autologous platelet gel in pain control and blood loss in total knee arthroplasty. An analysis of the haemoglobin, narcotic requirement and range of motion. Int Orthop 2007;31(3):309–13.

37. Zavadil DP, Satterlee CC, Costigan JM, et al. Autologous platelet gel and platelet-poor plasma reduce pain with total shoulder arthroplasty. J Extra Corpor Technol 2007;39(3):177–82.

38. Peerbooms JC, de Wolf GS, Colaris JW, et al. No positive effect of autologous platelet gel after total knee arthroplasty. Acta Orthop 2009;80(5):557–62.

39. Martin L, Auge C, Boue J, et al. Thrombin receptor: an endogenous inhibitor of inflammatory pain, activating opioid pathways. Pain 2009;146(1–2):121–9.

40. Sutter WW, Kaneps AJ, Bertone AL. Comparison of hematologic values and transforming growth factor-beta and insulin-like growth factor concentrations in platelet concentrates obtained by use of buffy coat and apheresis methods from equine blood. Am J Vet Res 2004;65(7):924–30.

41. Schnabel LV, Mohammed HO, Miller BJ, et al. Platelet rich plasma (PRP) enhances anabolic gene expression patterns in flexor digitorum superficialis tendons. J Orthop Res 2007;25(2):230–40.

42. Schnabel LV, Sonea HO, Jacobson MS, et al. Effects of platelet rich plasma and acellular bone marrow on gene expression patterns and DNA content of equine suspensory ligament explant cultures. Equine Vet J 2008;40(3):260–5.

43. McCarrel T, Fortier L. Temporal growth factor release from platelet-rich plasma, trehalose lyophilized platelets, and bone marrow aspirate and their effect on tendon and ligament gene expression. J Orthop Res 2009;27(8):1033–42.

44. Anitua E, Andia I, Sanchez M, et al. Autologous preparations rich in growth factors promote proliferation and induce VEGF and HGF production by human tendon cells in culture. J Orthop Res 2005;23(2):281–6.

45. Doucet C, Ernou I, Zhang Y, et al. Platelet lysates promote mesenchymal stem cell expansion: a safety substitute for animal serum in cell-based therapy applications. J Cell Physiol 2005;205(2):228–36.

46. Zhang J, Wang JH. Platelet-rich plasma releasate promotes differentiation of tendon stem cells into active tenocytes. Am J Sports Med 2010;38(12):2477–86.

47. Martineau I, Lacoste E, Gagnon G. Effects of calcium and thrombin on growth factor release from platelet concentrates: kinetics and regulation of endothelial cell proliferation. Biomaterials 2004;25(18):4489–502.

48. Textor JA, Norris JW, Tablin F. Effects of preparation method, shear force, and exposure to collagen on release of growth factors from equine platelet-rich plasma. Am J Vet Res 2011;72(2):271–8.

49. Spang JT, Tischer T, Salzmann GM, et al. Platelet concentrate vs. saline in a rat patellar tendon healing model. Knee Surg Sports Traumatol Arthrosc 2011;19(3): 495–502.

50. Lyras DN, Kazakos K, Verettas D, et al. The effect of platelet-rich plasma gel in the early phase of patellar tendon healing. Arch Orthop Trauma Surg 2009; 129(11):1577–82.

51. Aspenberg P, Virchenko O. Platelet concentrate injection improves Achilles tendon repair in rats. Acta Orthop Scand 2004;75(1):93–9.

52. Virchenko O, Grenegard M, Aspenberg P. Independent and additive stimulation of tendon repair by thrombin and platelets. Acta Orthop 2006;77(6):960–6.

53. Kajikawa Y, Morihara T, Sakamoto H, et al. Platelet-rich plasma enhances the initial mobilization of circulation-derived cells for tendon healing. J Cell Physiol 2008;215(3):837–45.

54. Murray MM, Spindler KP, Ballard P, et al. Enhanced histologic repair in a central wound in the anterior cruciate ligament with a collagen-platelet-rich plasma scaffold. J Orthop Res 2007;25(8):1007–17.

55. Bir SC, Esaki J, Marui A, et al. Angiogenic properties of sustained release platelet-rich plasma: characterization in-vitro and in the ischemic hind limb of the mouse. J Vasc Surg 2009;50(4):870–9, e872.

56. Bosch G, Moleman M, Barneveld A, et al. The effect of platelet-richplasma on the neovascularization of surgically created equine superficial digital flexor tendon lesions. Scand J Med Sci Sports 2010. DOI: 10.1111/j.1600-0838.2009.01070.x.

57. Lyras DN, Kazakos K, Verettas D, et al. The influence of platelet-rich plasma on angiogenesis during the early phase of tendon healing. Foot Ankle Int 2009; 30(11):1101–6.

58. Lyras DN, Kazakos K, Agrogiannis G, et al. Experimental study of tendon healing early phase: is IGF-1 expression influenced by platelet rich plasma gel? Orthop Traumatol Surg Res 2010;96(4):381–7.

59. Saito M, Takahashi KA, Arai Y, et al. Intraarticular administration of platelet-rich plasma with biodegradable gelatin hydrogel microspheres prevents osteoarthritis progression in the rabbit knee. Clin Exp Rheumatol 2009;27(2):201–7.

60. Milano G, Sanna Passino E, Deriu L, et al. The effect of platelet rich plasma combined with microfractures on the treatment of chondral defects: an experimental study in a sheep model. Osteoarthritis Cartilage 2010;18(7):971–80.

61. de Vos RJ, Weir A, van Schie HT, et al. Platelet-rich plasma injection for chronic Achilles tendinopathy: a randomized controlled trial. JAMA 2010; 303(2):144–9.

62. Schepull T, Kvist J, Norrman H, et al. Autologous platelets have no effect on the healing of human achilles tendon ruptures: a randomized single-blind study. Am J Sports Med 2011;39(1):38–47.

63. Bosch G, van Schie HT, de Groot MW, et al. Effects of platelet-rich plasma on the quality of repair of mechanically induced core lesions in equine superficial digital flexor tendons: a placebo-controlled experimental study. J Orthop Res 2010; 28(2):211–7.

64. Alvarez ME, Giraldo CE, Carmona JU. Monitoring bacterial contamination in equine platelet concentrates obtained by the tube method in a clean laboratory environment under three different technical conditions. Equine Vet J 2010; 42(1):63–7.

65. Tablin F, Walker NJ, Hogle SE, et al. Assessment of platelet growth factors in supernatants from rehydrated freeze-dried equine platelets and their effects on fibroblasts in vitro. Am J Vet Res 2008;69(11):1512–9.

66. Monteiro SO, Lepage OM, Theoret CL. Effects of platelet-rich plasma on the repair of wounds on the distal aspect of the forelimb in horses. Am J Vet Res 2009;70(2):277–82.

67. Hu H, Forslund M, Li N. Influence of extracellular calcium on single platelet activation as measured by whole blood flow cytometry. Thromb Res 2005;116(3): 241–7.

68. Murray MM, Forsythe B, Chen F, et al. The effect of thrombin on ACL fibroblast interactions with collagen hydrogels. J Orthop Res 2006;24(3):508–15.

69. Johnstone IB. Comparative effects of phenylbutazone, naproxen and flunixin meglumine on equine platelet aggregation and platelet factor 3 availability in vitro. Can J Comp Med 1983;47(2):172–9.

70. Spindler KP, Imro AK, Mayes CE, et al. Patellar tendon and anterior cruciate ligament have different mitogenic responses to platelet-derived growth factor and transforming growth factor beta. J Orthop Res 1996;14(4):542–6.

71. Balavoine JF, de Rochemonteix B, Williamson K, et al. Prostaglandin E2 and collagenase production by fibroblasts and synovial cells is regulated by urine-derived human interleukin 1 and inhibitor(s). J Clin Invest 1986;78(4):1120–4.

72. Hannum CH, Wilcox CJ, Arend WP, et al. Interleukin-1 receptor antagonist activity of a human interleukin-1 inhibitor. Nature 1990;343(6256):336–40.

73. Arend WP, Welgus HG, Thompson RC, et al. Biological properties of recombinant human monocyte-derived interleukin 1 receptor antagonist. J Clin Invest 1990; 85(5):1694–7.

74. Kato H, Ohashi T, Matsushiro H, et al. Molecular cloning and functional expression of equine interleukin-1 receptor antagonist. Vet Immunol Immunopathol 1997;56(3–4):221–31.

75. Frisbie DD, Ghivizzani SC, Robbins PD, et al. Treatment of experimental equine osteoarthritis by in vivo delivery of the equine interleukin-1 receptor antagonist gene. Gene Ther 2002;9(1):12–20.

76. Frisbie DD, Kawcak CE, Werpy NM, et al. Clinical, biochemical, and histologic effects of intra-articular administration of autologous conditioned serum in horses with experimentally induced osteoarthritis. Am J Vet Res 2007;68(3):290–6.

77. Morisset S, Frisbie DD, Robbins PD, et al. IL-1ra/IGF-1 gene therapy modulates repair of microfractured chondral defects. Clin Orthop Relat Res 2007;462:221–8.

78. Caron JP, Fernandes JC, Martel-Pelletier J, et al. Chondroprotective effect of intraarticular injections of interleukin-1 receptor antagonist in experimental osteoarthritis. Suppression of collagenase-1 expression. Arthritis Rheum 1996;39(9): 1535–44.

79. Chevalier X, Goupille P, Beaulieu AD, et al. Intraarticular injection of anakinra in osteoarthritis of the knee: a multicenter, randomized, double-blind, placebo-controlled study. Arthritis Rheum 2009;61(3):344–52.

80. Rutgers M, Saris DB, Dhert WJ, et al. Cytokine profile of autologous conditioned serum for treatment of osteoarthritis, in vitro effects on cartilage metabolism and intra-articular levels after injection. Arthritis Res Ther 2010;12(3):R114.
81. Meijer H, Reinecke J, Becker C, et al. The production of anti-inflammatory cytokines in whole blood by physico-chemical induction. Inflamm Res 2003;52(10): 404–7.
82. Arend WP. Interleukin-1 receptor antagonist: discovery, structure and properties. Prog Growth Factor Res 1990;2(4):193–205.
83. Seckinger P, Williamson K, Balavoine JF, et al. A urine inhibitor of interleukin 1 activity affects both interleukin 1 alpha and 1 beta but not tumor necrosis factor alpha. J Immunol 1987;139(5):1541–5.
84. Baragi VM, Renkiewicz RR, Jordan H, et al. Transplantation of transduced chondrocytes protects articular cartilage from interleukin 1-induced extracellular matrix degradation. J Clin Invest 1995;96(5):2454–60.
85. Larrick JW. Native interleukin 1 inhibitors. Immunol Today 1989;10(2):61–6.
86. Dinarello CA, Thompson RC. Blocking IL-1: interleukin 1 receptor antagonist in vivo and in vitro. Immunol Today 1991;12(11):404–10.
87. Fleischmann R, Stern R, Iqbal I. Anakinra: an inhibitor of IL-1 for the treatment of rheumatoid arthritis. Expert Opin Biol Ther 2004;4(8):1333–44.
88. Bondeson J, Blom AB, Wainwright S, et al. The role of synovial macrophages and macrophage-produced mediators in driving inflammatory and destructive responses in osteoarthritis. Arthritis Rheum 2010;62(3):647–57.
89. Calich AL, Domiciano DS, Fuller R. Osteoarthritis: can anti-cytokine therapy play a role in treatment? Clin Rheumatol 2010;29(5):451–5.
90. Malemud CJ. Anticytokine therapy for osteoarthritis: evidence to date. Drugs Aging 2010;27(2):95–115.
91. Yang KG, Raijmakers NJ, van Arkel ER, et al. Autologous interleukin-1 receptor antagonist improves function and symptoms in osteoarthritis when compared to placebo in a prospective randomized controlled trial. Osteoarthritis Cartilage 2008;16(4):498–505.
92. Baltzer AW, Moser C, Jansen SA, et al. Autologous conditioned serum (Orthokine) is an effective treatment for knee osteoarthritis. Osteoarthritis Cartilage 2009;17(2):152–60.
93. Pelletier JP, Caron JP, Evans C, et al. In vivo suppression of early experimental osteoarthritis by interleukin-1 receptor antagonist using gene therapy. Arthritis Rheum 1997;40(6):1012–9.
94. Daheshia M, Yao JQ. The interleukin 1beta pathway in the pathogenesis of osteoarthritis. J Rheumatol 2008;35(12):2306–12.

Stem Cell–based Therapies for Bone Repair

Peter I. Milner, BVetMed, PhD, CertES(Orth), MRCVS[a,*],
Peter D. Clegg, MA, Vet MB, PhD[a],
Matthew C. Stewart, BVSc, MVetClinStud, PhD[b]

KEYWORDS
• Stem cell • Bone repair • Osteogenesis • Horse

The use of cell-based therapies for bone repair in large animal orthopaedics has traditionally been through autologous bone grafts,[1] particularly in fracture fixation and arthrodesis techniques but also in other applications, such as the treatment of bone cysts.[2,3] Problems such as tissue loss, poor healing, high stress loads, and infection are important factors affecting outcomes in large animal orthopaedics.[4] To some degree, these areas have been addressed over the years with advances in surgical techniques, improved implant design, and local antibiotic delivery. However, because of these ongoing concerns, there has been considerable interest in the use of cell-based strategies for manipulating and improving bone repair. However, an appreciation of the biology behind bone healing is fundamental to understanding how and where cell-based therapy can be an adjunct to clinical bone repair.

OSTEOGENESIS AT THE SITE OF BONE REPAIR

After a fracture of a bone occurs, the mechanisms activated to effect bone repair are analogous to the development and formation of bone in early life (osteogenesis). The main difference is that fracture healing is usually preceded by an inflammatory response and subsequent increase in blood supply to the region. An understanding of the processes occurring in osteogenesis can provide important information with respect to the molecular and cellular events occurring in repair. This information emphasizes the importance of the cellular response to healing and therefore lends credence to the use of osteoprogenitor cells to enhance bone healing.

The authors have nothing to disclose.
[a] Department of Musculoskeletal Biology, University of Liverpool, Leahurst Campus, Chester High Road, Neston, Cheshire, CH64 7TE, UK
[b] Department of Veterinary Clinical Medicine, College of Veterinary Medicine, University of Illinois, 1008 West Hazelwood Drive, Urbana, IL 61802, USA
* Corresponding author.
E-mail address: p.i.milner@liverpool.ac.uk

Vet Clin Equine 27 (2011) 299–314
doi:10.1016/j.cveq.2011.05.002
0749-0739/11/$ – see front matter. © 2011 Elsevier Inc. All rights reserved.
vetequine.theclinics.com

Bone repair represents a series of overlapping phases, similar to most wound healing processes, including an inflammatory phase, a reparative phase, and a remodeling phase.[5] The inflammatory phase usually lasts for the first 2 to 3 weeks after injury and cellular responses are activated to begin the bone repair process and protect the healing tissue from infection. Cellular recruitment initially leads to replacement of the fracture hematoma with fibrous tissues and, progressively, cartilaginous matrix. As stability of the fracture site is increased, the cartilaginous matrix template is replaced by bone through endochondral ossification in both the periosteal and endosteal callus, resulting in interfragmentary stabilization (**Fig. 1**). Following bony bridging of the fracture site, in a period of months and years, the remodeling phase becomes dominant with osteonal remodeling occurring to continually replace and vascularize the new bone.

Recruitment of mesenchymal stromal cells (MSCs) to the fracture site is critical in bone repair. These cells reside in the bone marrow in low densities (comprising approximately 1 in 100 000 bone marrow cells).[6] Other sources of stromal cells include endosteal and periosteal osteoprogenitors, and circulating monocyte populations. Following an appropriate chemotactic stimulus, circulating stem cells home to a site of injury and contribute to repair mechanisms.

Within the fracture bed, many of the signaling pathways (including Indian hedgehog [Ihh], bone morphogenetic protein [BMP], and canonical wnt-β-catenin pathways) and transcription factors (including Runx2 and vascular endothelial growth factor [VEGF]) active during embryonic osteogenesis are also involved in cellular recruitment and differentiation in the repair process.[5–9] Osteoblastic differentiation of stromal cells is stimulated predominately by Wnt signaling, which upregulates the key osteogenic transcription factor, Runx2, and osteoblastic-specific genes such as *osteocalcin* and *collagen type 1* (**Fig. 2**).[10,11] Although Runx2 is involved in chondrocytic differentiation,[12] particularly in cell maturation at the growth plate,[13] it seems to be the master regulator that commits progenitor cells to the osteoblastic lineage. Furthermore, interaction with other osteoblastic signaling pathways, mediated by BMPs, Ihh, and activating transcription factor 4 (ATF4), are important for tissue maturation.[5] In addition to the resident stromal cell population, recent studies in adults have shown a small (1%) subpopulation of circulating monocytic cells that are capable of osteoblastic activities,[14] and these may be recruited to the fracture site through pathways such as the CXCR4/stromal cell–derived factor-1 chemotactic pathway.[15]

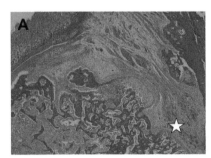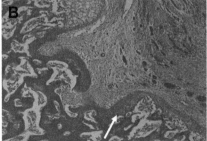

Fig. 1. Hematoxylin and eosin sections of rat femoral fracture callus ($\times 20$, $\times 40$). (*A*) Influx of blood vessels and fibrous tissue (*star*) can be seen between the disrupted ends of the trabecular bone. (*B*) At the front of the invading bone repair unit, osteoid (organic bone matrix) production by osteoblasts derived from MSCs can be seen (*arrow*). (Images *Courtesy of* Udo Hetzel, Department of Pathology, School of Veterinary Science, University of Liverpool, UK.)

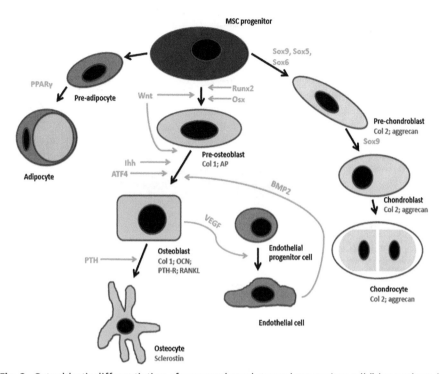

Fig. 2. Osteoblastic differentiation of a mesenchymal stromal progenitor cell (blue pathway). Stimulatory factors are shown in green. Gene products are shown in red. ATF4, activating transcription factor 4; BMP2, bone morphogenetic protein 2; col 1, collagen type 1; Col 2, collagen type 2; Ihh, Indian hedgehog; OCN, osteocalcin; Osx, osterix; PPARγ, peroxisome proliferator–activated receptor γ; PTH, parathyroid hormone; PTH-R, parathyroid hormone–receptor; RANKL, receptor activator of nuclear factor κ-B ligand; Runx2, runt-related transcription factor 2; Sox5, 6, and 9, SRY sex determining region Y (SRY)-box 5, 6, and 9; wnt, wingless and int signaling pathway.

Hypoxia and vascular disruption at the fracture site serve as additional stimuli to cellular differentiation and bone regeneration (**Fig. 3**). Neovascularization is a critical process required for fracture repair, and the application of exogenous VEGF has been shown to enhance bone formation.[16] The influx of blood vessels to the fracture site can occur through preexisting vessels (angiogenesis) as well as mobilization of circulating CD34+ endothelial progenitor cells (EPCs).[17] EPCs can directly participate in neovascularization as well as contributing to fracture repair in a paracrine fashion by secreting growth factors such as BMPs, VEGF, and FGF2 at the fracture site.[18] These factors secreted by EPCs can stimulate further growth factor release by osteoblasts.[19] In addition, the local hypoxic environment at the fracture site results in nuclear stabilization of the transcription factor HIF-1α, thereby leading to upregulation of HIF-responsive genes such as VEGF, further enhancing neovascularization and bone repair.[20]

The ability of stromal cells to survive and contribute to bone repair is dependent on factors such as fragment stability, vascularization, expression of growth factors, and other cellular factors. The fracture bed is a different environment from that present during normal bone development and the presence of ongoing inflammation and hypoxia provide additional challenges to these osteoprogenitor cells to contribute to

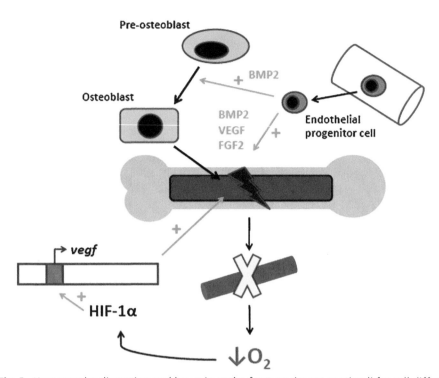

Fig. 3. How vascular disruption and hypoxia at the fracture site act as stimuli for cell differentiation and neovascularization. Following fracture, vascular disruption and inflammation occur, leading to hypoxia at the fracture bed. These processes act as stimuli for mobilization of circulating endothelial progenitor cells that can take part directly in neovascularization as well as contributing to the repair process in a paracrine fashion by influencing osteoblast differentiation. In addition, hypoxia results in nuclear stabilization of the transcription factor, HIF-1α and HIF-1α act on promoter regions upstream of genes containing hypoxic-responsive elements, such as *vegf*, to increase expression. BMP2, bone morphogenetic protein 2; FGF2, fibroblast growth factor 2; HIF-1α, hypoxia-inducible factor-1α.

the ultimate goal of bone repair. Clinical strategies that minimize fracture site inflammation and support rapid neovascularization, in turn, facilitate osteoprogenitor cell responses and accelerate repair.

CELL-BASED THERAPY FOR BONE REPAIR

Stem cells have the potential to differentiate into many different cell types in the body, and this characteristic has led to great excitement in human and veterinary medicine for the potential of stem cells to regenerate injured tissue.[21–25] In equine orthopaedics, the main focus of research and application has been the use of cells to augment tendon healing.[26] In large animal orthopaedics, cell-based therapies have been used for many years to aid fracture healing, primarily in the form of bone grafts,[2] but recent research has focused on the use of alternative cell-based applications to assist bone repair. Many of these techniques involve protection and delivery of stem cells to the fracture site, the use of genetically modified cells that express osteogenic factors, and the use of materials/drugs to recruit and modulate resident stem cell activity at the fracture site.

Bone Grafts

Many of the current techniques to assist bone repair in large animal orthopaedics involve the use of bone grafts. Autologous bone grafts are the current gold standard for stimulating bone formation in defects because they contain both osteogenic cells and osseous matrix.[19] Cancellous bone grafts contain a mix of cell subpopulations including fully differentiated osteoblasts as well as undifferentiated MSCs. These MSCs can respond to local environmental stimuli and differentiate into the required cell type(s), but these cells are present at low numbers in graft material and require a rigid environment containing the correct growth factor cues to survive and proliferate. It is believed that up to 90% of cells within bone grafts are lost during the grafting procedure.[2] Common sites for retrieval of bone graft in the horse include the sternum, tuber coxae, and proximal tibia.[27] In a study by McDuffee and Anderson,[28] the tuber coxae and tibial periosteum appeared to provide the largest quantities of viable osteoprogenitor cells.[28] It is advisable that bone grafts should be transported directly to the implantation site at the time of surgery, or temporarily stored in blood-soaked sponges, to reduce the risk of cell loss.

The main functions of bone grafts are osteoinduction and osteoconduction.[2,21] Osteoinduction refers to the induction of bone formation, whereas osteoconduction describes the physical support the graft material provides, as a scaffold, to facilitate new bone growth. Bone matrix, particularly the organic component, acts as an osteoinductive agent by delivering growth factors and cytokines such as BMPs and TGF-β that act as local chemotactants and stimulants for cell differentiation. The use of acellular demineralized bone matrix as osteoinductive grafts has been described in equine orthopaedics,[29] although, in an equine rib-defect model, demineralized bone matrix appeared to affect normal mineralization in a negative fashion compared with autologous cancellous bone grafts.[30]

Direct Application of MSCs for Bone Repair

MSCs have the ability to proliferate and differentiate into bone, cartilage, adipose, and muscle cells and have been used experimentally and clinically as an attractive method to augment bone repair. Freshly isolated and culture-expanded cells have been directly implanted into defects, leading to positive effects on clinical outcome. The direct injection of fresh bone marrow aspirates into bone defects has the distinct advantage of direct application at the time of primary surgical intervention but there are concerns about cell loss during transplantation, particularly with the low numbers of bone marrow stromal cells recovered by primary aspiration, compared with expanded populations, and the lack of a vehicle to retain the cells at the fracture site if injected alone. Accepting these concerns, the injection of freshly aspirated samples seems to have a positive benefit in the clinical environment and has been used, for example, to aid healing of tibial nonunion fractures in people.[31,32] Aspirates can be directly injected as unprocessed agents or concentrated at the bench-side before implantation. The latter strategy increases the concentration of stromal cells within the aspirate (by around 7 times)[33] but adds an additional step and time element to the preparation. In the study by Cuomo and colleagues,[33] bone marrow aspirate and mesenchymal stem cell–enriched bone marrow aspirate (each mixed with demineralized bone matrix) both resulted in bone repair in a rat femoral bone-defect model. No significant difference in bone volume produced was noted between the 2 methods, or between the 2 treatment groups and a control group containing demineralized bone matrix only, as assessed by radiographic healing and total bone volume. The quality of the repair using either bone marrow aspirate or mesenchymal stem cell–enriched bone marrow aspirate showed wide variability and both were inferior to groups treated with rhBMP-2 protein. This study also highlighted the considerable interindividual variability that can be expected in clinical applications of biologic therapies such as bone marrow aspirates.

Clonal expansion methods can generate increased numbers of undifferentiated cells and there are several reviews describing isolation and expansion techniques.[34–36] Clonal expansion requires the acquisition of stromal cells to initiate the procedure. As a consequence, such applications may have limitations in acute fracture management. Bone marrow is the classic source of MSCs where stromal cells from bone marrow aspirates are expanded before reimplantation days or weeks later. Bone marrow aspiration is straightforward to perform in the equid[37] but, in humans, is often associated with donor site morbidity and pain. The use of adipose-derived MSCs offers an alternative source of cells that is associated with fewer complications.[38] Equine adipose-derived MSCs have been shown to have both osteogenic and chondrogenic capacities.[39] Other osteoprogenitor cell sources include blood[40–42] and umbilical cord cells.[43–45] Once the initial stromal cell population has been expanded to a clinically suitable level (approximately 1×10^7 cells/mL), implantation into the bone defect can be performed; again, cell retention at the surgical site may be compromised if implantation is not supported by an effective vehicle or scaffold.

To improve osteogenic differentiation of MSCs, pharmacologic manipulation can be applied to alter gene expression and stimulate production of osteogenic factors. Several of these approaches are based on current understanding of osteogenic differentiation and cell commitment during normal skeletogenesis, and many of the recognized pathways have been investigated as potential targets for bone formation and repair. The parathyroid hormone (PTH) analog teriparatide (1-34 PTH), developed as a treatment of osteoporosis, upregulates osterix and Runx2 gene expression in MSCs in a murine fracture model, accelerating osteogenic commitment and increasing fracture callus size in treated animals.[46] PTH-based drugs have also been shown to enhance mechanical strength in adult rat fractures in vivo.[47] In an equine diaphyseal cortical-defect model, the implantation of human 1-34 PTH gene-activated matrix increased periosteal bone formation compared with controls (untreated defect in contralateral limb),[48] although PTH matrix implantation did not improve the repair of concurrently induced subchondral bone defects. The use of a 1-34 PTH–enriched fibrin hydrogel has been described in the resolution of a subchondral cystic lesion in the proximal interphalangeal joint of a horse following transosseous curettage,[49] although the extent to which the PTH hydrogel contributed to bone healing in this case is not clear.

MSC response to growth factors, particularly BMPs, can result in alterations in osteogenic differentiation. BMPs (particularly BMP-2), and VEGF administration stimulate MSC proliferation and increase the production of osteogenic factors.[50] The effects of other growth factors differ between studies; for example, IGF-1 has been shown to both stimulate and inhibit osteogenic differentiation in separate studies.[50,51] This may be caused by the temporal and spatial effects of growth factors on a biologic process that can be difficult to replicate in vitro.[50] Modulation of Wnt signaling seems to affect the growth and osteogenic differentiation of MSCs.[52] The induced expression of Dickkopf-1 (Dkk-1), an inhibitor of the canonical Wnt pathways, inhibited osteogenesis, whereas the glycogen synthetase-β inhibitor, LiCl, accelerated osteogenesis.[53] Other pathways that can be regulated to stimulate bone formation include the cAMP/protein kinase A (PKA) pathway as shown by the finding that upstream PKA activators lead to osteogenic gene induction and enhanced bone production in human MSCs.[54] It is clear from these studies that understanding the signaling pathways involved in osteogenesis is important because these could provide new classes of pharmacologic agents used for the enhancement of bone repair.

EPCs and Bone Repair

EPCs are nonmesenchymal cells that can contribute to bone repair by secreting growth factors and modulating cell differentiation and behavior at the fracture site.[55] These cells can originate from bone marrow as well as migrating, albeit in low numbers, from the circulating population of peripheral monocytes. Following fracture, these CD34+ cells are mobilized from the bone marrow into the circulation and are then recruited to the fracture site to contribute to endothelial cell differentiation.[18] EPCs secrete angiogenic factors such as VEGF in a paracrine fashion and therefore contribute to fracture site healing, particularly neovascularization.[17] Recently, several groups have implanted CD34+ cells isolated from peripheral blood into fracture models and have shown enhanced bone healing. In an ovine tibial-defect model, EPCs implanted into a critical-sized gap stimulated formation of dense woven bone throughout the defect after 8 to 12 weeks, compared with fibrotic scar tissue in the sham-operated group.[56] In a similar study using a rat segmental femoral defect, repairs in the EPC treatment group also showed evidence of complete union.[57] From these experimental results, it seems that local EPC, in addition to MSC applications, could prove to be an effective cell-based treatment of bone repair.

Use of Scaffolds and Other Biomaterials to Enhance Cell-based Bone Repair

As discussed earlier, protection and support of implanted cells is important for cell survival and consequent biologic contributions to bone repair. There is increasing interest in the use of cells seeded onto biodegradable scaffolds or other materials for bone tissue engineering, based on their ability to contribute to osteogenesis. The basic requirements of bioscaffolds relate to biocompatibility, mechanical properties, and the ability to biodegrade in a predictable manner. Scaffolds need to function in a supportive role to allow cell attachment and proliferation and subsequent extracellular matrix (ECM) deposition. Scaffolds have traditionally been seen as biologically passive, having a structural role, whereas more recently developed scaffold constructs are increasingly able to influence cell osteogenesis and matrix deposition. Altering the material properties of these compounds can itself affect bone repair independently of any contribution from implanted cells.[58] The value of autologous MSCs seeded onto ceramic scaffolds has been assessed in various models of bone loss (nonunion) or bone formation (spinal fusion). In an ovine critical tibial-defect model, the use of cell-loaded scaffolds accelerated bone repair.[59] Similarly, implants loaded with autologous stem cells showed increased bone deposition in a canine critical-sized segmental femoral defect.[60]

Several studies have investigated the use of β-tricalcium phosphate (β-TCP) as a biocompatible scaffold (**Fig. 4**).[61,62] Calcium phosphate–based matrices seeded with MSCs are able to promote osteoblastic-specific marker expression[63] and recently it has been shown that β-TCP matrix can trigger the osteogenic differentiation of adipose-derived stem cells.[64] Calcium phosphate and chitosan constructs seeded with human umbilical cord mesenchymal stem cells have been used for craniofacial reconstruction, showing increased bone mineral synthesis[65] compared with the scaffold substrate alone. The use of a polylactic acid/β-TCP composite in a three-dimensional matrix also enhanced osteogenic differentiation of adipose-derived stem cells,[66] as measured by alkaline phosphatase and osteocalcin levels, without the need for osteogenic media supplementation. Although β-TCP has good osteoconductive properties,[67] it has low compressive strength and a rapid resorption rate, and these properties limit its use as a load-bearing scaffold.[68]

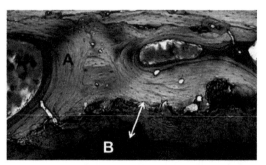

Fig. 4. Osteoconduction by β-tricalcium phosphate. The ceramic coating of the metallic prosthesis (B) is indicated by the double-ended arrow. Direct apposition and integration of bone (A) onto the ceramic surface is clearly evident.

Bioglass, glass-ceramic, and bioceramics containing CaO and SiO_2 possess apatite-formation ability in body fluid and exhibit good bioactivity as bone implant materials. Ceramics containing Ca^{2+}, Mg^{2+}, and Si, such as akermanite ($Ca_2MgSi_2O_7$), seem to have a more controlled degradation rate compared with β-TCP and can closely bond with bone tissue when implanted. Importantly for cell-based therapy, they also seem to enhance osteogenic differentiation of seeded bone marrow stromal cells,[69] possibly through surface formation of apatite crystals and the consequent release of bioactive ions.[70]

In addition to calcium phosphate and other ceramic-based scaffolds, other materials have been assessed for their ability to support and differentiate stem cells in bone repair. Cell-seeded porous poly(ε-caprolactone) (PCL) scaffolds showed significantly higher bone ingrowth and torsional strength in a nude rat critical-sized femoral-defect model compared with femora receiving scaffolds alone,[71] although consistent bridging of the defect was not observed, possibly because of the lack of long-term retention of live cells at the defect site. Oh and colleagues[72] showed that MSC osteogenesis was enhanced by interaction with titanium oxide (TiO_2) nano-tubes. In subsequent work, this group showed that MSC response was a consequence of the unique nanotopographic properties and high biocompatibility of the TiO_2 surface and was influenced by the nanotube dimensions.[73] Tubes between 70 and 100 nm resulted in stem cell elongation and selective differentiation into osteoblastlike cells and appeared to influence osseous integration. The material properties of titanium metal make it ideal for bone biologic applications. Concurrently optimizing the nanotopographic characteristics of these constructs promotes the most favorable conditions for osteogenic cells and is important for their therapeutic efficacy.

Cell-based Gene Therapy for Bone Repair

Cell-based gene therapy offers the ability to deliver cells that have been manipulated to selectively express key osteogenic factors to fracture and nonunion sites,[74] which provides an efficient mechanism for long-term release of factors to enhance bone repair. Adult MSCs have been engineered to deliver BMP-2, BMP-4, and BMP-9 to promote osteogenic differentiation and bone formation in murine models.[75,76] Genetically engineered MSCs also have the advantage that they can be integrated into the damaged tissue while expressing these genes during a prolonged period of time, compared with a single administration of expression constructs or proteins to the repair site.[61] The use of MSCs rather than non-MSCs to express osteogenic factors has additional advantages: it seems that MSCs become fully integrated into the bone cortex, whereas, when non-MSCs are used, the cells remain as discrete bone-forming units with no continuity within the bone.[77] Other regulatory factors, such as VEGF, when expressed at fracture sites using modified MSCs, lead to a synergistic effect on bone production when coexpressed with BMP-4.[78] Zachos and colleagues[79] augmented osteogenic differentiation in equine bone marrow–derived MSCs using adenoviral delivery of BMP-2 and BMP-6. In addition to MSCs from the bone marrow niche, other sources of stem cells, such as muscle and adipose tissues, have also been used for the delivery of gene therapy to bone.[80,81]

One significant concern regarding gene therapy is that this approach may lead to overexpression of these factors and consequent overproduction of bone, which in itself may be undesirable. One method to address this concern is to link gene expression to a drug-regulated promoter such as tetracycline or doxycycline, where expression of the osteogenic gene can be turned on or off by administration of the drug.[82] However, these regulatory systems do not provide complete control of gene expression; incomplete activation and/or inactivation of expression is common because other cell factors may indirectly influence promoter activity, and construct silencing following genomic integration limits expression longevity.[83] In addition, because the implantation of non–genetically modified MSCs results in increased osteogenesis, it raises the question of whether genetic modification of MSCs is necessary for clinical efficacy. Further research needs to be done to determine whether increasing the expression of key osteogenic factors can substantively enhance MSC osteogenic differentiation and improve the ability to manage large bone defects.

The Periosteum as a Source of Osteoprogenitor Cells in Bone Repair

The periosteum is a well-recognized source of osteoprogenitor cells and growth factors in bone healing and has often been undervalued as a source of repair cells in comparison with blood and/or bone marrow. Osteoprogenitors are located within the inner cellular or cambium periosteal layer, immediately adjacent the bone surface. The outer periosteal cell layer is fibrous in nature. Periosteal osteoprogenitors are far more numerous in young animals than in adults (**Fig. 5**), a factor that contributes to the marked age-dependent differences in fracture repair rates. Creation of a space between the periosteum and parent bone generates large quantities of new bone in a rabbit model.[84] In a critical-sized ovine femoral-defect model, the periosteum was used as a sleeve to surround a missing section of bone, resulting in bridging bone formation across the defect that did not occur in controls.[85] Indeed, periosteal isogenic allografting of bone defects in mice showed that up to 70% of the graft-derived osteogenesis was associated with expansion and differentiation of donor periosteal progenitor cells because removal of periosteum resulted in a sharp decrease in bone cartilaginous callus formation.[86]

Recently, the molecular pathways that regulate periosteal mesenchymal cell differentiation have been investigated. Wang and colleagues[87] showed that the endogenous expression of BMP-2 by periosteal cells was critical in periosteal-mediated callus formation at the onset of healing. In a separate study, the same group isolated early periosteal callus-derived MSCs and showed that activation of the hedgehog (Hh) signaling pathway was important in promoting osteogenic and chondrogenic differentiation.[88] These studies highlight the importance of the periosteum as a source of osteoprogenitor cells for bone repair and also emphasize the potential value of engineering a functional periosteum to enhance the reparative properties of allografts or bone substitutes for bone repair.[89]

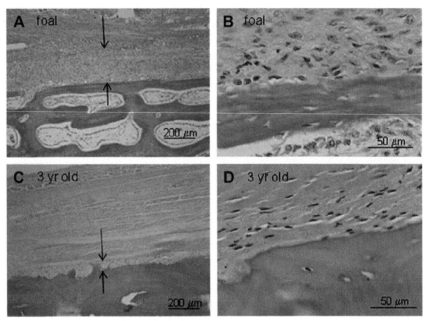

Fig. 5. Periosteal osteoprogenitors. The inner cell layer (cambium) of periosteum in a foal (*A, B*) and an adult horse (*C, D*) is indicated between the opposed arrows in *A* and *C*. Under higher magnification (*B, D*), the difference in cellularity of the osteoprogenitor populations immediately adjacent the bone surface is clearly evident. (Images *Courtesy of* David Coleman, Department of Pathobiology, College of Veterinary Medicine, University of Illinois.)

Noninvasive Assessment of Stem Cells in Bone Healing

Measurement of bone tissue properties following implantation is important when determining the success of particular treatments, particularly in relation to stem cell applications in bone repair. Both invasive and noninvasive methods of assessing bone repair have been described. Invasive methods, although superior to noninvasive assays, usually involve sacrifice of the experimental animal; therefore, for clinical scenarios, noninvasive methods are preferable.

Radiography can provide a crude index of bone repair but microcomputed tomography has been used to quantify trabecular bone volume, distribution, and morphology in bone regenerates and mineralized matrix formation within biomaterials, both in vitro and in vivo.[90,91] Selection of the radiograph attenuation threshold can be used to detect mineralized ECM within low-attenuating materials such as scaffolds and thereby assess bone deposition from differentiated osteoprogenitor cells. In addition to mineral deposition, vascular ingrowth can also be assessed by this method.[92,93]

Labeling cells with quantum dots (QDs) is a method commonly used for in vivo cell labeling and tracking. Cells internalize the fluorescent semiconductor nanocrystals without apparent effect on cell viability or function,[94] although one study suggested that inhibition of hMSC osteogenesis was caused by QD labeling.[95] Toxicity is a potential concern with QDs; QDs are usually composed of a cadmium-selenium core surrounded by a biologically insert zinc sulfide shell, and degradation of the shell may result in expose to toxic cadmium. In a study by Dupont and colleagues,[71] QD-labeled stem cells could be visualized in a segmental defect for up to 7 to 10 days after implantation; beyond this interval, QD signals also appeared at other sites, because of the movement of macrophages containing endocytosed QDs from the immediate defect site. Other in vivo tracking techniques have been developed that may assist in monitoring cell fate. These techniques include transduction of green fluorescent protein expression cassettes and cell labeling with magnetic iron oxide nanoparticles that can be detected by MRI.[96–98]

SUMMARY

The use of stem cell therapy in bone repair has considerable potential for clinical application in the horse, although currently such therapies have not progressed much beyond the use of cancellous bone grafts. The use and manipulation of stromal cells (and others such as EPCs) to stimulate osteogenesis are logical steps to improve bone repair, but this approach may still be limited in large animal orthopaedics because of the need for immediate applications, particularly for fracture fixation. The banking of osteoprogenitor cells on appropriate scaffolds may be a potential way around this problem. Whatever the solution, it is likely that cell-based therapy will, at some stage, provide important additional treatment options for bone repair in equine orthopaedic surgery.

REFERENCES

1. von Rechenberg B, Auer JA. Bone grafts and bone replacements. In: Auer JA, Stick JA, editors. Equine surgery. St Louis (MO): WB Saunders; 2006. p. 1030–6.
2. Jackson WA, Stick JA, Arnoczky SP, et al. The effect of compacted cancellous bone grafting on the healing of subchondral bone defects of the medial femoral condyle in horses. Vet Surg 2000;29(1):8–16.
3. Fortier LA, Nixon AJ. New surgical treatments for osteochondritis dissecans and subchondral bone cysts. Vet Clin North Am Equine Pract 2005;21(3):673–90.
4. Richardson DW. Complications of orthopaedic surgery in horses. Vet Clin North Am Equine Pract 2009;24(3):591–610.
5. Deschaseaux F, Sensebe L, Heymann D. Mechanisms of bone repair and regeneration. Trends Mol Med 2009;15(9):417–29.
6. Clines GA. Prospects for osteoprogenitor stem cells in fracture repair and osteoporosis. Curr Opin Organ Transplant 2010;15(1):73–8.
7. Bruder SP, Fink DJ, Caplan AI. Mesenchymal stem cells in bone development, bone repair and skeletal regeneration therapy. J Cell Biochem 1994;56(3): 283–94.
8. Reddi AH. Bone and cartilage differentiation. Curr Opin Genet Dev 1994;4(5): 737–44.
9. Rosen V. BMP2 signaling in bone development and repair. Cytokine Growth Factor Rev 2009;20(5–6):475–80.
10. Yamaguchi A, Komori T, Suda T. Regulation of osteoblast differentiation mediated by bone morphogenetic proteins, hedgehogs and Cbfa1. Endocr Rev 2000;21(4): 393–411.
11. Qi H, Aguiar D, Williams SM, et al. Identification of genes responsible for osteoblast differentiation from human mesodermal progenitor cells. Proc Natl Acad Sci U S A 2003;100(6):3305–10.
12. Fujita T, Azuma Y, Fukuyama R, et al. Runx2 induces osteoblast and chondrocytes differentiation and enhances their migration by coupling with PI3K-Akt signaling. J Biol Chem 2004;166(1):85–95.
13. Enomoto H, Enomoto-Iwamoto M, Iwamoto M, et al. Cbfa1 is a positive regulatory factor in chondrocyte maturation. J Biol Chem 2000;275(12):8695–702.

14. Eghbali-Fatourechi GZ, Lamsam J, Fraser D, et al. Circulating osteoblast-lineage cells in humans. N Engl J Med 2005;352(19):1959–66.

15. Otsuru S, Tamai K, Yamazaki T, et al. Circulating bone marrow-derived osteoblast progenitor cells are recruited to the bone-forming site by the CXCR4/stromal cell-derived factor-1 pathway. Stem Cells 2008;26(1):223–34.

16. Street J, Bao M, deGuzman L, et al. Vascular endothelial growth factor stimulates bone repair by promoting angiogenesis and bone turnover. Proc Natl Acad Sci U S A 2002;99(15):9656–61.

17. Lee DY, Cho TJ, Kim JA, et al. Mobilisation of endothelial progenitor cells in fracture healing and distraction osteogenesis. Bone 2008;42(5):932–41.

18. Matsumoto T, Mifune Y, Kawamoto A, et al. Fracture induced mobilization and incorporation of bone marrow-derived endothelial progenitor cells for bone healing. J Cell Physiol 2008;215(1):234–42.

19. Deckers MM, van Bezooijen RL, van der Horst G, et al. Bone morphogenetic proteins stimulate angiogenesis through osteoblast-derived vascular endothelial growth factor A. Endocrinology 2002;143(4):1545–53.

20. Wan C, Gilbert SR, Wang Y, et al. Activation of the hypoxia-inducible factor-1alpha pathway accelerates bone regeneration. Proc Natl Acad Sci U S A 2008;105(2):686–91.

21. Kraus KH, Kirker-Head C. Mesenchymal stem cells and bone regeneration. Vet Surg 2006;35(3):232–42.

22. Zaidi N, Nixon AJ. Stem cell therapy in bone repair and regeneration. Ann N Y Acad Sci 2007;1117:62–72.

23. Waese EY, Kandel RR, Stanford WL. Application of stem cells in bone repair. Skeletal Radiol 2008;37(7):601–8.

24. Nourissat G, Diop A, Maurel N, et al. Mesenchymal stem cell therapy regenerates the native bone-tendon junction after surgical repair in a degenerative rat model. PLoS One 2010;5(8):e12248.

25. Derubeis AR, Cancedda R. Bone marrow stromal cells (BMSCs) in bone engineering: limitations and recent advances. Ann Biomed Eng 2004;32(1):160–5.

26. Smith RK. Mesenchymal stem cell therapy for equine tendinopathy. Disabil Rehabil 2008;30(20–22):1752–8.

27. Boero MJ, Schneider JE, Mosier JE, et al. Evaluation of the tibia as a source of autogenous cancellous bone in the horse. Vet Surg 1989;18(4):322–7.

28. McDuffee LA, Anderson GI. In vitro comparison of equine cancellous bone graft donor sites and tibial periosteum as sources of viable osteoprogenitors. Vet Surg 2003;32(5):455–63.

29. Fackelman GE, von Rechenberg B, Fetter AW. Decalcified bone grafts in the horse. Am J Vet Res 1981;42(6):943–8.

30. Kawcak CE, Trotter GW, Powers BE, et al. Comparison of bone healing by demineralized bone matrix and autogenous cancellous bone in horses. Vet Surg 2000;29(3):218–26.

31. Connolly JF, Guse R, Tiedeman J, et al. Autologous marrow injection as a substitute for operative grafting of tibial nonunions. Clin Orthop Relat Res 1991;266:259–70.

32. Hernigou P, Poignard A, Manicom O, et al. The use of percutaneous autologous bone marrow transplantation in nonunion and avascular necrosis of bone. J Bone Joint Surg Br 2005;87(7):896–902.

33. Cuomo AV, Virk M, Petrigliano F, et al. Mesenchymal stem cell concentration and bone repair: potential pitfalls from bench to bedside. J Bone Joint Surg Am 2009;91(5):1073–83.

34. Gregory CA, Prockop DJ, Spees JL. Non-haematopoietic bone marrow stem cells: molecular control of expansion and differentiation. Exp Cell Res 2005;306(2): 330–5.

35. Delorme B, Charbord P. Culture and characterization of human bone marrow mesenchymal stem cells. Methods Mol Med 2007;140:67–81.

36. Gnecchi M, Melo LG. Bone marrow-derived mesenchymal stem cell: isolation, expansion, characterisation, viral transduction, and production of conditioned medium. Methods Mol Biol 2009;482:281–94.

37. Smith RK, Korda M, Blunn GW, et al. Isolation and implantation of autologous equine mesenchymal stem cells from bone marrow into the superficial digital flexor tendon as a potential novel treatment. Equine Vet J 2003;35(1):99–102.

38. Lindroos B, Suuronen R, Miettinen S. The potential of adipose stem cells in regenerative medicine. Stem Cell Rev 2011;7(2):269–91.

39. Braun J, Hack A, Weis-Klemm M, et al. Evaluation of the osteogenic and chondrogenic differentiation capacities of equine adipose tissue-derived mesenchymal stem cells. Am J Vet Res 2010;71(10):1228–36.

40. Zvaifler NJ, Marinova-Mutafchieva L, Adams G, et al. Mesenchymal precursor cells in the blood of normal individuals. Arthritis Res 2000;2(6):477–88.

41. Clarke AD, Jørgensen HG, Mountford J, et al. Isolation and therapeutic potential of human haematopoietic stem cells. Cytotechnology 2003;41:111–31.

42. Jones E, McGonagle D. Human bone marrow mesenchymal stem cells in vivo. Rheumatology 2008;47:126–31.

43. Lee MW, Choi MS, Yang YJ, et al. Mesenchymal stem cells from cryopreserved human umbilical cord blood. Biochem Biophys Res Commun 2004;320:273–8.

44. Lu LL, Liu YJ, Yang SG, et al. Isolation and characterisation of human umbilical cord mesenchymal stem cells with haematopoiesis-supportive function and other potentials. Haematologica 2006;91(8):1017–26.

45. Toupadakis CA, Wong A, Geneto DC, et al. Comparison of the osteogenic potential of equine mesenchymal stem cells from bone marrow, adipose tissue, umbilical cord blood, and umbilical cord tissue. Am J Vet Res 2010;71(10):1237–45.

46. Kaback LA, Soung do Y, Naik A, et al. Teriparatide (1–34 human PTH) regulation of osterix during fracture repair. J Cell Biochem 2008;105(1):219–26.

47. Andreassen TT, Willick GE, Morley P, et al. Treatment with parathyroid hormone hPTH(1–34), hPTH(1–31), and monocyclic hPTH(1–31) enhances fracture strength and callus amount after withdrawal fracture strength and callus mechanical quality continue to increase. Calcif Tissue Int 2004;74:351–6.

48. Backstrom KC, Bertone AL, Wisner ER, et al. Response of induced bone defects in horses to collagen matrix containing the human parathyroid hormone gene. Am J Vet Res 2004;65(9):1223–32.

49. Fuerst A, Derungs S, von Rechenberg B, et al. Use of a parathyroid hormone peptide (PTH(1–34))-enriched fibrin hydrogel for the treatment of a subchondral cystic lesions in the proximal interphalangeal joint of a warmblood filly. J Vet Med A Physiol Pathol Clin Med 2007;54(2):107–12.

50. Huang Z, Nelson ER, Smith RL, et al. The sequential expression profiles of growth factors from osteoprogenitors to osteoblasts in vitro. Tissue Eng 2007;13:2311–20.

51. Yeh LC, Lee JC. Co-transfection with the osteogenic protein (OP)-1 gene and the insulin-like growth factor (IGF)-I gene enhanced osteoblastic cell differentiation. Biochim Biophys Acta 2006;1763:57–63.

52. Gregory CA, Gunn WG, Reyes E, et al. How Wnt signaling affects bone repair by MSCs from bone marrow. Ann N Y Acad Sci 2005;1049:97–106.

53. Gregory CA, Perry AS, Reyes E, et al. Dkk-1-derived synthetic peptides and lithium chloride for the control and recovery of adult stem cells from bone marrow. J Biol Chem 2005;280(3):2309–23.
54. Siddappa R, Martens A, Doorn J, et al. cAMP/PKA pathway activation in human mesenchymal stem cells in vitro results in robust bone formation in vivo. Proc Natl Acad Sci U S A 2008;105(2):7281–6.
55. Khosla S, Westendorf JJ, Mödder UL. Concise review: insights from normal bone remodelling and stem cell-based therapies foe bone repair. Stem Cells 2010; 28(12):2124–8.
56. Rozen N, Bick T, Bajayo A, et al. Transplanted blood-derived endothelial progenitor cells (EPC) enhance bridging of sheep tibia critical size defects. Bone 2009; 45(5):918–24.
57. Atesok K, Li R, Stewart DJ, et al. Endothelial progenitor cells promote fracture healing in a segmental bone defect model. J Orthop Res 2010;28(8):1007–14.
58. Yuan H, Fernandes H, Habibovic P, et al. Osteoinductive ceramics as a synthetic alternative to autologous bone grafting. Proc Natl Acad Sci U S A 2010;107(31): 13614–9.
59. Kon E, Muraglia A, Corsi A, et al. Autologous bone marrow stromal cells loaded onto porous hydroxyapatite ceramic accelerate bone repair in critical-size defects of sheep long bones. J Biomed Mater Res 2000;49(3):328–37.
60. Arinzeh TL, Peter SJ, Archambault MP, et al. Allogenic mesenchymal stem cells regenerate bone in a critical-sized canine segmental defect. J Bone Joint Surg Am 2003;85(10):1927–35.
61. LeGeros RZ. Properties of osteoconductive biomaterials: calcium phosphates. Clin Orthop Relat Res 2002;395:81–98.
62. Arinzeh TL, Tran T, Mcalary J, et al. A comparative study of biphasic calcium phosphate ceramics for human mesenchymal stem-cell-induced bone formation. Biomaterials 2005;26:3631–8.
63. Muller P, Bulnheim U, Diener A, et al. Calcium phosphate surfaces promote osteogenic differentiation of mesenchymal stem cells. J Cell Mol Med 2008;12(1): 281–91.
64. Marino G, Rosso F, Cafiero G, et al. Beta-tricalcium phosphate 3D scaffold promote alone osteogenic differentiation of human adipose stem cells: in vitro study. J Mater Sci Mater Med 2010;21(1):353–63.
65. Xu HH, Zhao L, Weir MD. Stem cell-calcium phosphate constructs for bone engineering. J Dent Res 2010;89(12):1482–8.
66. Haimi S, Suuriniemi N, Haaparanta AM, et al. Growth and differentiation of adipose stem cells on PLA/bioactive glass and PLA/beta-TCP scaffolds. Tissue Eng Part A 2009;15(7):1473–80.
67. Rose PL, Auer JA, Hulse D, et al. Effect of beta-tricalcium phosphate in surgically created subchondral bone defects in male horses. Am J Vet Res 1988;49(3): 417–24.
68. Tanimoto Y, Nishiyama N. Preparation and physical properties of tricalcium phosphate laminates for bone-tissue engineering. J Biomed Mater Res A 2008;85(2): 427–33.
69. Sun H, Wu C, Dai K, et al. Proliferation and osteoblastic differentiation of human bone marrow-derived stromal cells on akermanite-bioactive ceramics. Biomaterials 2006;27(33):5651–7.
70. Wu C, Chang J, Ni S, et al. In vitro bioactivity of akermanite ceramics. J Biomed Mater Res A 2006;76(1):73–80.

71. Dupont KM, Sharma K, Stevens HY, et al. Human stem cell delivery for treatment of large segmental bone defects. Proc Natl Acad Sci U S A 2010;107(8):3305–10.
72. Oh SH, Finones RR, Daraio C, et al. Growth of nano-scale hydroxyapatite using chemically treated titanium oxide nanotubes. Biomaterials 2005;26(24):4938–43.
73. Oh SH, Brammer KS, Li YS, et al. Stem cell fate dictated solely by altered nanotube dimensions. Proc Natl Acad Sci U S A 2009;106(7):2130–5.
74. Gafni Y, Turgeman G, Liebergal M, et al. Stem cells as vehicles for orthopedic gene therapy. Gene Ther 2004;11(4):417–26.
75. Lieberman JR, Daluiski A, Stevenson S, et al. The effect of regional gene therapy with bone morphogenetic protein-2-producing bone-marrow cells on the repair of segmental femoral defects in rats. J Bone Joint Surg Am 1999;81(7):905–17.
76. Wright V, Peng H, Usas A, et al. BMP4-expressing muscle-derived stem cells differentiate into osteogenic lineage and improve bone healing in immunocompetent mice. Mol Ther 2002;6(2):169–78.
77. Gazit D, Turgeman G, Kelly P, et al. Engineered pluripotent mesenchymal cells integrate and differentiate in regenerating bone: a novel cell mediated gene therapy. J Gene Med 1999;1(2):121–33.
78. Peng H, Wright V, Usas A, et al. Synergistic enhancement of bone formation and healing by stem cell-expressed VEGF and bone morphogenetic protein-4. J Clin Invest 2002;110(6):751–9.
79. Zachos TA, Shields KM, Bertone AL. Gene-mediated osteogenic differentiation of stem cells by bone morphogenetic proteins-2 or -6. J Orthop Res 2006;24(6):1279–91.
80. Musgrave DS, Pruchnic R, Bosch P, et al. Human skeletal muscle cells in ex vivo gene therapy to deliver bone morphogenetic protein-2. J Bone Joint Surg Br 2002;84(1):120–7.
81. Dragoo JL, Choi JY, Lieberman JR, et al. Bone induction by BMP-2 transduced stem cells derived from human fat. J Orthop Res 2003;21(4):622–9.
82. Hasharoni A, Helm GA, Gazit D, et al. Murine spinal fusion induced by engineered mesenchymal stem cells that conditionally express bone morphogenetic protein-2. J Neurosurg Spine 2005;3(1):47–52.
83. Rang A, Will H. The tetracycline-responsive promoter contains functional interferon-inducible response elements. Nucleic Acids Res 2000;28(5):1120–5.
84. Stevens MM, Marini RP, Schaefer D, et al. In vivo engineering of organs: the bone bioreactor. Proc Natl Acad Sci U S A 2005;102(32):11450–5.
85. Knothe Tate ML, Ritzman TF, Schneider E, et al. Testing of a new one-stage bone-transport surgical procedure exploiting the periosteum for the repair of long-bone defects. J Bone Joint Surg Am 2007;89(2):307–16.
86. Zhang X, Xie C, Lin AS, et al. Periosteal progenitor cell fate in segmental cortical bone graft transplantations: implication for functional tissue engineering. J Bone Miner Res 2005;20(12):2124–37.
87. Wang Q, Huang C, Xue M, et al. Expression of endogenous BMP-2 in periosteal progenitor cells is essential for bone healing. Bone 2011;48(3):524–32.
88. Wang Q, Huang C, Zeng F, et al. Activation of the Hh pathway in periosteum-derived mesenchymal stem cells induces bone formation in vivo: implication for post-natal bone repair. Am J Pathol 2010;177(6):3100–11.
89. Zhang X, Awad HA, O'Keefe RJ, et al. A perspective: engineering periosteum for structural bone graft healing. Clin Orthop Relat Res 2008;466(8):1777–87.
90. Jones AC, Milthorpe B, Averdunk H, et al. Analysis of 3D bone ingrowth into polymer scaffolds via micro-computed tomography imaging. Biomaterials 2004;25(20):4947–54.

91. Oliveira AL, Malafaya PB, Costa SA, et al. Micro-computed tomography (micro-CT) as a potential tool to assess the effect of dynamic coating routes on the formation of biomimetic apatite layers on 3D-plotted biodegradable polymeric scaffolds. J Mater Sci Mater Med 2007;18(2):211–23.
92. Guldberg RE, Ballock BD, Boyan CL, et al. Analyzing bone, blood vessels and biomaterials with microcomputed tomography. IEEE Eng Med Biol Mag 2003; 22(5):77–83.
93. Guldberg RE, Duvall CL, Peister A, et al. 3D imaging of tissue integration with porous biomaterials. Biomaterials 2008;29(28):3757–61.
94. Shah BS, Clark PA, Moioli EK, et al. Labeling of mesenchymal stem cells by bioconjugated quantum dots. Nano Lett 2007;7(10):3071–9.
95. Hsieh SC, Wang FF, Lin CS, et al. The inhibition of osteogenesis with human bone marrow mesenchymal stem cells by Cd Se/ZnS quantum dot labels. Biomaterials 2006;27(8):1656–64.
96. Kawanami A, Matsushita T, Chan YY, et al. Mice expressing GFP and CreER in osteochondroprogenitor cells in the periosteum. Biochem Biophys Res Commun 2009;386(3):477–82.
97. Kanczler JM, Sura HS, Magnay J, et al. Controlled differentiation of human bone marrow stromal cells using magnetic nanoparticle technology. Tissue Eng Part A 2010;16(10):3241–50.
98. Jing X, Yang L, Duan X, et al. In vivo MR imaging tracking of magnetic iron oxide nanoparticle labeled, engineered, autologous bone marrow mesenchymal stem cells following intra-articular injection. Joint Bone Spine 2008;75(4):432–8.

Cell-based Therapies for Tendon and Ligament Injuries

A.G.L. Alves, DVM, MS, PhD[a], Allison A. Stewart, DVM, MS[b],
J. Dudhia, PhD[c], Y. Kasashima, DVM, PhD[d],
A.E. Goodship, BVSc, PhD, MRCVS[e],
R.K.W. Smith, MA, VetMB, PhD, DEO, MRCVS[c,*]

KEYWORDS

• Equine • Stem cell • Regenerative therapy • Tendon healing

Overstrain and traumatic tendon and ligament injuries are common in the horse and, for the most part, heal (repair) naturally by the formation of scar tissue. However, the scar tissue formed in this repair is functionally deficient compared with normal tendon, which has important consequences for the animal in terms of reduced performance and a substantial risk of reinjury, despite the multitude of treatments that have been proposed. Regenerative medicine offers the prospect of restoring normal, or close to normal, structure and function to an injured organ, thereby resulting in a successful restoration of activity without the risk of reinjury. Regenerative medicine aims to harness the combined effects of a cell source, scaffold support, and anabolic stimulus to facilitate the healing of the injury.[1]

There are multiple choices for the selection of a cell source for regenerative medicine, and at this time it is not clear which source will prove to be therapeutically optimal. A logical source of cells for making new tendon tissue would be the tenocytes

Disclosures: R.K.W.S. is a technical adviser of VetCell.
Experimental work has been funded by the Horserace Betting Levy Board, VetCell, and the Japan Racing Association and has been performed in collaboration with Prof Allen Goodship, Prof Peter Clegg, Dr Jayesh Dudhia, Dr Yoshi Kasashima, Dr Debbie Guest, Dr Sandra Strassberg, and Dr Lucy Richardson.

[a] Department of Veterinary Surgery and Anesthesiology, School of Veterinary Medicine and Animal Science, São Paulo State University, Botucatu, São Paulo 18618970, Brazil
[b] Department of Veterinary Clinical Medicine, College of Veterinary Medicine, University of Illinois, 1008 West Hazelwood Drive, Urbana, IL 61802, USA
[c] Department of Veterinary Clinical Sciences, The Royal Veterinary College, University of London, Hawkshead Lane, North Mymms, Hatfield, Hertfordshire, AL9 7TA, UK
[d] Clinical Science and Pathology Division, Equine Research Institute, Japan Racing Association, 321-4, Tokami-cho, Utsunomiya, Tochigi, Japan
[e] Institute of Orthopaedics and Musculoskeletal Science, University College London, Royal National Orthopaedic Hospital, Stanmore, Middlesex, HA7 4LP, UK
* Corresponding author.
E-mail address: rksmith@rvc.ac.uk

Vet Clin Equine 27 (2011) 315–333
doi:10.1016/j.cveq.2011.06.001
0749-0739/11/$ – see front matter © 2011 Published by Elsevier Inc.

themselves. However, the biopsy of tendon to prepare and propagate cells leads to formation of a secondary lesion at the donor site, an unacceptable option for flexor tendons in the horse. In addition, cells derived from different tendons do show different characteristics in culture,[2] which may compromise their effectiveness when implanted into other tendons. Alternative sources of differentiated fibroblasts under investigation include dermal and ligament fibroblasts. Ligament fibroblasts not only have potential advantages in that they are often more metabolically active than other fibroblasts but also have different cell characteristics that may not be appropriate for use in tendon repair. However, the cells carrying the greatest hope for effective therapy are stem cells. Stem cells are defined as cells capable of differentiating into different cell lines and the 2 most studied are embryonic stem cells (ESCs; those derived from the embryo and capable of differentiating into every cell type in the body and therefore truly pluripotent) or mesenchymal stem cells (MSCs; those derived from postnatal tissues with multipotential capabilities to derive cells of mesenchymal origin). The terminology for these cells is not standardized and the terms mesenchymal stem, stromal, and progenitor cells are used interchangeably.

MSCs are generally found in varying but sparse numbers in many postnatal tissues and frequently reside as perivascular cells, whereby they likely play a role in normal turnover and tissue maintenance.[3] MSCs have been isolated from a wide variety of tissues, of which the most established sources are bone marrow and fat. Other sources potentially useful for tendon and ligament cell therapies include umbilical cord blood cells, which potentially span the divide between fetal and postnatal stem cells and therefore could have greater regenerative potential. Furthermore, they can be easily recovered at birth and stored for future use. However, although umbilical cord blood is a relatively rich source of hematopoietic stem cells, studies have not consistently shown that cord blood is a reliable source of MSCs, and considerably more work is needed in this area before these cells can be advocated for clinical use.[4,5] This article focuses on the use of stem cells derived from embryos, bone marrow, fat, and tendon and their potential for the treatment of tendon and ligament injuries.

FEATURES OF TENDON AND LIGAMENT INJURY THAT LEND ITSELF TO CELL THERAPY

Equine digital flexor tendon strain injuries provide many of the additional elements required for tendon tissue engineering. The lesion manifests within the central core of the tissue, thus providing a natural enclosure for implantation that, by the time of stem cell implantation, is filled with granulation tissue, which acts as a scaffold (**Fig. 1**). Tendon lesions have the added advantage of being highly vascularized and therefore capable of nutritional support to the implanted progenitor cells. The anabolic stimulus is provided by the cytokine and mechanical environment, which are potentially important stimuli for differentiation, in the intratendinous location of the cells and augmented by the suspension of MSCs in growth factor–rich solutions, such as bone marrow supernatant, which we have shown to have significant anabolic effects in vitro.[6]

Postinjury, tendon does not exhibit restrictions of cellular infiltration but those cells actually involved in the synthesis of new scar tissue are mostly locally derived cells.[4] Most tissues have a small population of precursor cells (tissue-specific progenitor cells) that function to replenish cells lost through natural turnover and aid in repair after injury. Evidence of multipotency has been shown for cells derived from young tendon[5,7]; however, in adult tendon, investigators have been unable to demonstrate the presence of a cell subpopulation capable of differentiating into multiple cell

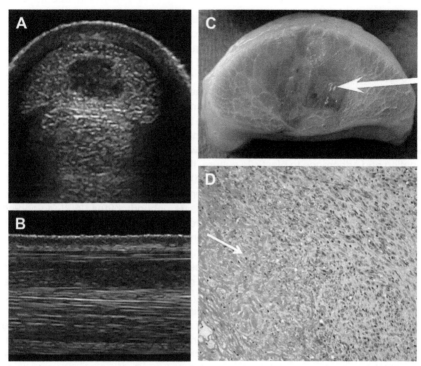

Fig. 1. Ultrasonographic, gross, and histologic appearances of superficial digital flexor tendinopathy. Transverse (*A*) and longitudinal (*B*) ultrasonographic images showing a central hypoechoic (core) lesion in the superficial digital flexor tendon. (*C*) Gross appearance of a healing core lesion (*arrow*). (*D*) Histologic appearance showing marked angiogenic response (*arrow*), marked cellular infiltration, and disorganized matrix structure during healing.

lineages (osteocytes, adipocytes, chondrocytes), as with bone marrow–derived cells. This limitation may explain why the influence of adult tendon progenitors in the repair process is restricted and results in natural repair inferior to normal tendon.

POTENTIAL THERAPEUTIC MECHANISMS OF STEM CELLS

The goal of using stem cells is to engineer new tendon tissue using cellular synthetic machinery. This goal can be achieved either via a direct contribution through differentiation into tissue-specific cell phenotypes and the production of tissue-appropriate extracellular matrix products or indirectly by trophic effects through the production of bioactive proteins, such as growth factors, antiapoptotic factors, and chemotactic agents.[8–10] In addition, recent studies have suggested an antiinflammatory role of implanted stem cells. Animal model studies have demonstrated that MSCs are hypoimmunogenic and inhibit the activation of T and B lymphocytes and natural killer cells.[11,12] The precise mechanism of the antiinflammatory effect of these cells is largely unknown, although a combination of this activity along with an antiapoptotic effect, additional recruitment of local multipotent stem cells, stimulation of vascular ingrowth, and the liberation of growth factors could all contribute to tissue repair.[4,13,14] It is not known which of these actions occur after stem cell implantation, although current opinion favors the paracrine actions as being most important.[15]

Bone Marrow–Derived MSCs

Bone marrow contains a hematopoietic stem cell population, from which the cellular components of blood are derived, and a stromal network of fibroblastlike cells. Among these stromal cells, there is a subpopulation of multipotent cells, the MSCs,[16] that are able to generate mesenchyme, the mass of tissue that develops mainly from the mesoderm of the embryo. These MSCs represent a small fraction of the total population of nucleated cells in bone marrow from human beings and cats, and only 0.001% to 0.01% of mononuclear cells isolated from a Ficoll density gradient of bone marrow aspirate are MSCs; this is presumed to be similar in horses.[17]

Bone marrow–derived MSCs have been shown to be multipotent. In addition to self-replication and adherence to plastic in culture, they are able to exhibit osteogenic, adipogenic, and chondrogenic differentiation with appropriate growth factor stimulus. Thus, the presence of MSCs is frequently demonstrated by the ability of a derived cell population to differentiate into osteoblasts, chondrocytes, and adipocytes, capable of producing bone, cartilage, and fat, respectively, in vitro. In addition to characterizing these cells by their ability to differentiate into distinct cell lineages, MSCs can be further characterized by cell surface markers.[18] However, their use in horses has been hampered because many of the positive stem cell markers described for other species use antibodies that show little or no cross-reactivity. The ability to select tendon tissue–promoting MSC populations by cell surface markers, with or without further modification, may be important for optimizing this therapy in the future.

We have chosen to harness the action of MSCs recovered from bone marrow because of ease of recovery and minimal donor site morbidity and, because these stem cells can be recovered from adult tissue, this source allows autologous reimplantation, which carries fewer regulatory and safety issues. Furthermore, in comparative experiments assessing multipotency, bone marrow–derived MSCs frequently outperform MSCs from other sources.[19–21] We have therefore hypothesized that the implantation of autologous MSCs, in far greater numbers than are present normally within tendon tissue, will improve the repair of the tendon both structurally, as shown by optimizing mechanical properties, organization, and composition, and functionally, as measured by reduced reinjury rates.

Technique for the recovery of bone marrow–derived stem cells

Bone marrow is recovered in heparinized containers from the sternum (or, less commonly, the tuber coxae) under standing sedation. Marrow aspiration is generally performed within 3 months of injury, when there is an enclosed area of disruption still visible ultrasonographically. The aspirate is transferred to a laboratory in specially designed containers for culture and expansion of MSCs, which yields an enriched rather than a pure cell preparation. After approximately 3 weeks, the cultured cells are shipped back to the veterinarian (usually 10×10^6 cells, although this dose is increased empirically up to 50×10^6 if lesions are very large) and implanted into the damaged tendon of the same horse under ultrasonographic guidance (**Fig. 2**). The cells are suspended in citrated bone marrow supernatant for implantation so that no foreign material (such as fetal bovine serum) is implanted and to gain potential beneficial effects of the rich mixture of growth factors present in the supernatant.[6]

Delivery, engraftment, and survival

We have shown in our laboratories that equine MSCs, cultured on fresh acellular equine tendon sections, not only survived, proliferated, and migrated into the matrix but also expressed extracellular matrix genes, although their expression was less than that of tenocytes cultured on the same tendon matrices.[22,23] Longer culture times

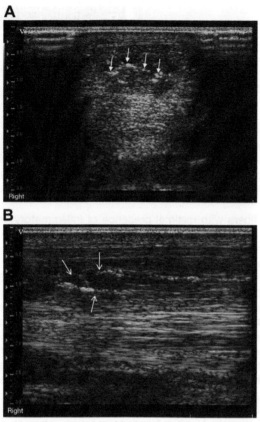

Fig. 2. Transverse (*A*) and longitudinal (*B*) ultrasonographs immediately after cell implantation showing the location of the injected cell suspension by the presence of air bubbles (*arrows*).

(3 weeks) resulted in greater similarities to tenocytes with MSCs lining up along the collagen fascicles. In vivo, we and others[4,24] have been able to demonstrate that the implanted cells survive within the tendon after implantation in relatively low numbers for up to 4 months (**Fig. 3**). However, although this technique allows high numbers to be delivered directly to the site of injury, it limits the use of the cells to distinct constrained lesions. To date, we are not able to treat contralateral tendons (which are likely to have a pathological condition but may not have a core lesion) or surface defects (eg, intrasynovial tendon tears). Intrasynovial administration may be an option for surface defects, and regional administration may also be possible, whereas systemic administration needs to address issues of homing to the injury site and engraftment.

Safety
The implantation of a cell type that is capable of self-renewal and had been implicated in the pathogenesis of certain cancers suggests a possible risk of neoplastic transformation. However, histopathologic examination of 17 tendons or ligaments from postmortem samples obtained from 12 horses that had undergone MSC implantation did not reveal any abnormal or neoplastic tissue. Instead, there was evidence of organized

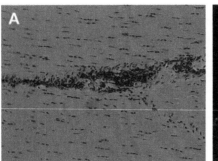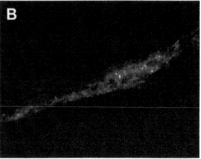

Fig. 3. Histologic (*A*) and fluorescence (*B*) images of MSCs after implantation into a damaged superficial digital flexor tendon. Note the retention of cells within the endotenon.

crimped collagen fibers with minimal presence of inflammatory cells. We have not conducted extensive postmortem examinations on tissues at remote sites (such as the lungs), but there have been no reports of clinically significant abnormalities of other body systems after implantation.

Reported adverse reactions after the treatment of more than 1500 clinical cases have been rare. Only 1 horse developed peritendinous mineralization 2 years after MSC implantation; this may have been related to the original trauma rather than a consequence of the cell implantation. Needle tracts are common in the first few months after implantation (**Fig. 4**), although it is unlikely that they adversely affect the outcome, given their focal nature; they usually resolve within 3 months. Gamma scintigraphy was performed 3 months after implantation in 6 horses but this did not demonstrate any bone formation within the treated tendons, suggesting that this is an unlikely consequence of MSC implantation.

Four further cases have experienced acute inflammatory reactions: one was mild and transient and thought to be a bandage reaction, whereas the other 3 cases were associated with intrasynovial administration, which is an off-label use for the preparation. It is possible that these 3 cases were the result of infection through contaminated bone marrow supernatant. An extra filtration step is now included in the preparation to minimize this risk.

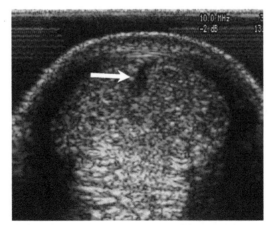

Fig. 4. Needle tracts (*arrow*) commonly found at follow-up ultrasound scans after implantation.

Efficacy

In vitro, MSCs cultured in 2- and 3-dimensional matrices can be induced to synthesize matrices with some of (but not all) the characteristics of tendon extracellular matrix. Equine MSCs can synthesize an abundant and remarkably well-structured matrix when cultured in vitro in a bioreactor within the coagulated supernatant of bone marrow. However, although several reliable determinants of osteogenic, adipogenic, and chondrogenic differentiation are available, demonstration of tenogenic differentiation is more problematic, partly because an effective tenogenic stimulus has not been well defined and fewer definitive tenocyte phenotypic markers have been identified. Tenocytes in culture have a fibroblastic morphology that is similar to MSCs and so cannot be identified from appearance alone. Collagen type I is the primary protein synthesized by tenocytes, but this does not distinguish these cells from fibroblasts capable of producing connective tissues, including scar tissue, in which deposition of collagen type III occurs in significant quantities. The synthesis of the glycoprotein cartilage oligomeric matrix protein (COMP) provides a more discriminating analysis but it too is not specific to tendon, although COMP does have a restricted distribution in tissues primarily designed to withstand load (eg, cartilage, tendon, and fibrocartilage). The use of a signature profile of synthesized extracellular matrix proteins enables a better discrimination between most musculoskeletal tissues. In addition, the transcription factor scleraxis and the transmembrane protein tenomodulin[25] are selectively expressed by partially differentiated mesenchymal precursors of connective tissue and tendon; these might therefore be indicative markers of the tenocyte lineage.[26] New markers of tendon differentiation will add to our ability to identify tenocyte lineages.

In vivo, MSCs have been implanted into surgically created tendon defects in multiple in vivo experiments using laboratory animal models, with almost universally positive outcomes. Most of these studies used surgically created defects in rabbit or rat tendons and have showed variable regeneration of new tendonlike tissue in defects implanted with MSCs in a biodegradable scaffold (collagen gel, Vicryl (polyglactin 910; Ethicon, Summerville, NJ) knitted mesh, or fibrin glue) as assessed by histology or simple biochemical assays.[27–30] However, not all have shown an improvement in microstructure, and, because allogenic cells were implanted, an inflammatory reaction persisted. Furthermore, the implanted cells exhibited a fibroblastic morphology but were not fully characterized as tenocytes. In more recent studies, MSC implantation was associated with both improved strength and quality of reparative tissue (determined by collagen type I/collagen type III ratio).[31] Thus, MSC-seeded constructs implanted in vivo are able to integrate into the tissue and synthesize tissue-specific extracellular matrix; however, it is unclear which factors are initiating this functional differentiation.

Although it is possible to demonstrate that implanted cells do survive, it has not yet been possible to demonstrate that the implanted cells actually synthesize, or induce the synthesis of, a tendonlike matrix or identify the mechanisms of these effects. Furthermore, it is not clear whether such a mechanism may arise from a truly regenerative response or whether any benefit arises more from an influence on the inflammatory process that follows injury. Recently, experimental studies in horses using a collagenase-induced injury have demonstrated significant improvements in some, but not all, parameters.[32–34] A surgical model[35] is as an alternative to test cell therapies, although initial data have not shown a significant effect on collagen fibril diameter (C.J. Caniglia, M.C. Schramme and R.K.W. Smith, unpublished data, 2011). However, in a controlled study of MSC versus saline treatments in naturally occurring tendinopathy in horses, mechanical testing and biochemical and molecular analyses of the new tissue synthesized after treatment demonstrated that stem cell treatment seemed to improve histologic scores of the healing tissue toward that of normal tendon compared with saline injection (Young and colleagues, unpublished data, 2011).

Ultrasonographic appraisal of treated cases show a rapid filling in of hypoechoic lesions, although the longitudinal striated pattern of the regenerated tendon rarely returns completely to normal (**Fig. 5**). In the analysis of 113 racehorses treated with bone marrow–derived MSCs, the reinjury percentage was 27.4%, with the rate for flat (n = 8) and National Hunt (n = 105) racehorses being 50% and 25.7%, respectively.[36] This recurrence rate was significantly less than those published for National Hunt racehorses treated in other ways (P<.05 vs Ref.[37]; P<.01 vs Ref.[38]). No relationship between outcome and age, discipline, number of MSCs injected, and injury to implantation interval was identified. In further support of this improved outcome, reinjury rates in sports horses showed a similar reduction after MSC administration.

A more limited number of cases with injuries to other tendons and ligaments have been treated with bone marrow–derived MSCs. For lesions present within a tendon sheath, cell implantation is usually done after tenoscopic evaluation to ensure that there are no surface defects through which the cells could leak.

ESCs

ESCs carry the major hopes of stem cell science because of their seemingly unlimited capability to generate all functional adult cell types. Permanent ESC cell lines can be established and maintained in a pluripotent undifferentiated state. At the blastocyst stage of development, the preimplantation mammalian embryo separates into the inner cell mass (ICM) cells of the putative embryo and the trophectoderm cells that will eventually form the outermost layer of the fetal placenta. Appropriate

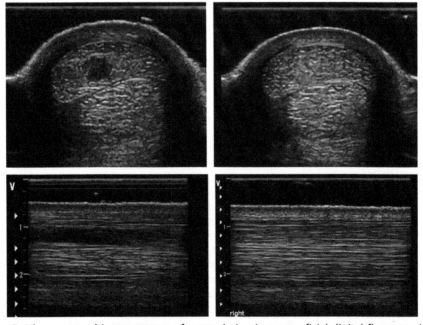

Fig. 5. Ultrasonographic appearance of a core lesion in a superficial digital flexor tendon treated with bone marrow–derived MSCs. There has been rapid filling in of the lesion, but the longitudinal pattern has not completely returned to normal.

environmental stimuli can cause ICM cells to differentiate into the cell types of all 3 germ layers: ectoderm, endoderm, and mesoderm, both in vitro and in vivo. Furthermore, it has become apparent that the culture requirements for proliferation and maintenance of ESCs in an undifferentiated state and the nature of the stimuli required to induce ESCs to transform into specialized end-stage cells of specific phenotype vary between humans and various animal species.[39,40] In addition, as genetic manipulations can be performed and confirmed in culture, ESCs have become a powerful tool for the generation of reporter cell lines or gain-of-function/loss-of-function disease models.[41–46]

Because the generation of ESC cell lines necessitates the destruction of an embryo, the development of these cells for clinical use has been associated with considerable ethical issues, especially in the human context. These issues may be, but are not necessarily, less ethically problematic for equine use. In an attempt to circumvent these issues, the exciting recent discovery of induced pluripotent stem (iPS) cells, derived from transfection of somatic (adult) cells with specific transcription factor genes, represents a possible alternative. iPS cells have been derived from equine cells,[41] but considerably more research is needed before these cells will be regulated sufficiently well to be used effectively and safely in clinical cases.

Use in horses

A recent study has reported the use of putative ESCs in the treatment of damaged equine flexor tendon.[4] In this study, the survival and distribution of ESCs were compared with those of MSCs. ESC persistence was higher than that of MSCs in the damaged superficial digital flexor tendon (SDFT), with numbers remaining at a constant level over 90 days. This could occur because the ESC population was either proliferating or was maintained by a balanced rate of proliferation and death, but it does suggest that ESCs respond positively to the tendon environment. Furthermore, the high survival rate of the ESCs coupled with minimal leukocyte infiltration suggests that the ESCs were not recognized as foreign by the host immune system. The different effects of ESCs and MSCs on tendon regeneration are not clear in this study, and future studies need to address which of these cell types will be of the most therapeutic benefit.

Although there are concerns that ESCs cannot be used for direct transplantation because of the risk of teratoma formation, no equine studies have reported this consequence.[4,39] The failure of equine ESC-like cells to generate teratomas in an immunoprivileged site could be an experimental failure or a peculiarity of equine ESCs. This finding remains difficult to explain, given that ESC implantation in other species, under similar conditions, produced teratomas.[39,47–49] It should also be stressed that teratoma formation at sites other than the implantation site in a very large animal and in a relatively short time frame is difficult to assess. Further investigation on the consequences of equine ESC transplantation is required to determine whether this anomaly is because of a peculiarity of equine pluripotent cells or because the ESC-like cells tested were not true ESCs.[50]

ESCs offer tremendous potential for regenerative therapy in tissues with an inherently limited capacity for self-repair. However, it is clear that more controlled studies are needed to show efficacy with respect to optimizing tendon and ligament repair to enable clinical use of ESCs with success.

Fat-Derived MSCs

Adipose tissue provides an alternative source of cells capable of multipotential differentiation. These cells have gained importance because adipose tissue is readily accessible in large quantities and adipose tissue–derived MSCs have been shown to be largely indistinguishable from bone marrow–derived MSCs. However, some studies have shown these cells to differentiate less capably into specific cell lineages.[19–21]

Technique for the recovery of fat-derived MSCs

Adipose tissues can be harvested from several sites in horses, including inguinal, sternal, and gluteal regions. The area over the dorsal gluteal muscles, at the base of the tail, is the most accessible in standing horses, and it can provide significant quantities of tissue, although there can be relatively little fat available in some highly athletically tuned thoroughbred racehorses. The horse is sedated, the area over the dorsal gluteal muscles is aseptically prepared, and skin and subcutaneous tissues are desensitized by local infiltration of 2% lidocaine using an inverted L-block. An incision of approximately 10 to 15 cm in length is made parallel to and approximately 15 cm abaxial to the vertebral column, exposing a layer of adipose tissue between the skin and musculature. Approximately 5 to 15 mL of adipose tissue can be harvested over the superficial gluteal fascia, and the skin incision is then sutured with nylon material.[14,21]

To isolate the cells, the adipose tissue is finely minced and digested with a collagenase solution prepared in a suitable tissue cultured medium. Tissue digestion can be performed over 3 to 6 hours or overnight (18 hours), depending on need and convenience. After digestion, the nucleated cell fraction is separated and concentrated. These adipose-derived nucleated cells (ADNCs) have been used immediately for injection into tendon lesions[13] or have been subjected to further expansion in cell culture, which may also enrich the stem cell fraction, similar to the technique used for bone marrow cells, before implantation as adipose-derived MSCs (AD-MSCs).[14]

It is important to recognize the difference between these 2 approaches. The nucleated cell fraction released from the adipose tissue, referred to as the stromal vascular fraction (SVF), is a mixed population of cells that includes endothelial cells and preadipocytes and a relatively low number of MSCs.[21] However, because SVFs have not been expanded in culture, they are termed minimally manipulated and are therefore subject to less regulatory issues in human medicine. In contrast, AD-MSCs expanded in the laboratory, although involving greater cost and labor, have the potential advantage that a greater number and a more homogeneous MSC population are generated. To date, there have been no reports of adverse consequences after ADNC administration, as opposed to a more purified stem cell preparation, although the relative therapeutic efficacies of these cell preparations have not been established. It is not apparent from the literature which of these preparations is preferable for tendon healing,[13] and there are no published studies evaluating the optimal number of AD-MSCs that should be used in the treatment of tendinitis. It is possible that optimization of the AD-MSC dose used in tendon therapy could improve the future results of such studies.[32]

Efficacy

There are only a few controlled studies investigating the use of AD-MSCs for the treatment of tendon injuries in horses. Analysis of the ultrasonographic appearance of the tendons revealed no significant differences between the ultrasonographic parameters of limbs that received AD-MSCs or ADNCs and their controls. Scores for linear collagen fiber pattern improved in both groups in these studies.[13,14] However, histologic scoring showed that the lesions treated by AD-MSCs were more organized and had a more uniform tissue repair compared with the control limbs, including lower cellularity in the tendon, less inflammatory infiltrate, lower fibroblastic density, greater parallel arrangement of the fibers, larger extracellular matrix deposits, and greater type I collagen expression.[13,14,16] However, no significant differences were evident in the immunohistochemical assessments of cell proliferation and type I collagen spatial organization, although there was a reduction in the formation of type III collagen in the tendons that received treatment.[13]

Expression of COMP was significantly increased in ADNC-injected tendons. Concentration of COMP in equine digital flexor tendons has been positively correlated with ultimate tensile strength and stiffness in young adult normal tendons, which suggests that COMP concentrations may be linked to organization of the tendon matrix.[51] This increase in expression of COMP messenger RNA (mRNA) in the ADNC-treated tendon could be related to the improvements in tendon architecture and, consequently, in tendon regeneration.[13]

Bone Marrow Aspirate

The first attempts to harness MSCs from bone marrow for the treatment of tendons and ligaments utilized the direct injection of neat bone marrow from the sternum.[52] This strategy was reported to be successful primarily for the treatment of suspensory ligament disease, although the outcomes were derived from an uncontrolled clinical case series. In this technique, bone marrow aspirate is collected from the sternum, followed by direct injection of relatively large volumes (usually 10–40 mL) of the heterogeneous mixed-cell population into the tendon/ligament lesion. If the aspiration is performed efficiently, anticoagulant is not necessary. This further simplifies the direct aspiration–injection approach. The advantages of this procedure are the simplicity of the technique, the ability to perform the procedure immediately at the time of diagnosis, and relatively low cost, but the disadvantage is the injection of a heterogeneous mixed-cell population, with few stem cells. Furthermore, there is some concern about the use of the bone marrow aspirate in tendons because of the potential for mineralization (**Fig. 6**), although this has not been reported to be a common finding by users of this technique. This technique has largely been superseded by more specific techniques designed to supply a more pure population and higher number of MSCs. Using a method analogous to the adipose tissue stem cell technique, the nucleated cell population from bone marrow (bone marrow mononuclear cell fraction [BMMNC]) or bone marrow aspirate concentrate can be recovered by centrifugation. These preparations have a reduced proportion of MSCs (and contain mainly white blood cells) but allow horse-side preparation that optimizes timing and cost of treatment.

The clinical effect of these cruder techniques might be due to bioactive substances in the noncellular fraction, such as growth factors produced by cells or platelets,[17] or the potential of the small number of MSCs or other cells.[21] The effect of BMMNC administration has been assessed in a collagenase-induced experimental model of tendon healing in horses[34] in which BMMNCs seemed to improve the deposition of certain extracellular matrix proteins such as type I collagen and COMP and reduce the levels of collagen type III, indicating scar tissue, compared with control horses. The response to BMMNC injection was similar to the response to cultured bone marrow–derived MSCs, although there were greater numbers of white blood cells retained in the tissue.

Tendon-Derived MSCs

Our work on tendon-derived stem cells is based on the rationale that cells derived from the target tissue/organ (in this case, tendon) will be phenotypically and biosynthetically more capable of stimulating tissue-specific functional repair than cells

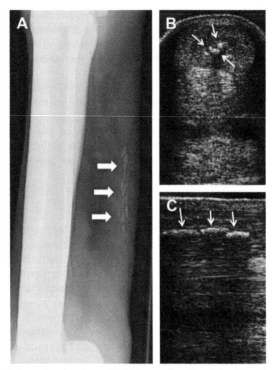

Fig. 6. Ossification/mineralization in an SDFT 7 months after injection of neat bone marrow. Note the scattered areas of radiodensity (*A; arrows*) and shadowing (*arrows*) seen in transverse (*B*) and longitudinal (*C*) ultrasonographic images.

isolated from distant sites. Tendon-derived MSCs have been isolated in humans, rats, and horses using a variety of isolation techniques, including cell migration from tendon explants, differential adherence of isolated cells, and MSC cell surface markers.[5,53,54] In humans, it has been estimated that 1 in every 10,000 cells isolated from tendon matrix are MSCs.[5]

Tendon-derived cells isolated using these techniques can differentiate along osteogenic, adipogenic, and chondrogenic lineages.[53,54] Equine tendon-derived cells have been isolated in our laboratory using a differential adherence technique developed for isolating skeletal muscle MSCs,[55] whereby the culture medium and unattached cells are serially transferred to fresh culture flasks every 12 to 24 hours over the first 72 hours of culture. Using this technique, 17 to 19 days are required for monolayer culture expansion through 2 passages, with an average yield of 7.9×10^6 cells.[22] Tendon-derived cells reach clinically relevant cell numbers (10 million cells) in a shorter period than bone marrow–derived cells. In addition, tendon-derived cells had higher cell viability and integrated better onto acellular tendon explants when compared with bone marrow–derived mesenchymal cells (**Fig. 7**)[22] and express higher levels of tendon extracellular matrix gene mRNAs.[56] In addition, tendon-derived cells had increased collagen and proteoglycan synthesis levels than bone marrow–derived cells. More recent studies have determined that supplementing monolayer cultures with basic fibroblast growth factor increases tendon-derived cell proliferation in monolayer,[56] providing a means to accelerate the generation of clinically useful numbers for reimplantation.

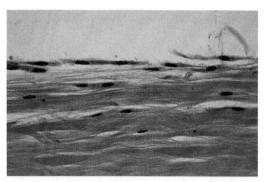

Fig. 7. Tendon-derived cells seeded on acellular tendon explants show linear distribution along the surface of the explants and some penetration into the underlying matrix (original magnification ×100).

Efficacy

We have assessed the clinical value of tendon-derived stem cell administration in the collagenase-induced SDFT model. Horses with collagenase-induced SDFT lesions were injected with tendon-derived progenitor cells in one forelimb and an equal volume of saline in the opposite forelimb 21 days after collagenase injections. The outcome analyses from this study are still ongoing, but there were no differences in total collagen content, total proteoglycan content, or ex vivo collagen and proteoglycan synthesis between the saline-treated and the tendon-derived progenitor cell–treated groups. However, both injured tendons had significantly increased collagen I, collagen III, COMP, and tenomodulin mRNA levels when compared with normal tendon. Histologically, the extracellular matrix organization of repair tissue in tendons treated with tendon-derived cells was closer to normal tendon than the saline-treated injured tendons. Specifically, there was a significant increase in the intensity of picrosirius red staining of fibrillar collagen and decreased proteoglycan staining (by toluidine blue) at the site of repair in tendons treated with tendon-derived cells, compared with controls (**Fig. 8**).

Tracking studies showed that tendon-derived progenitor cells stained with Dil were localized around the immediate injection site 1 week after administration, had migrated into the lesion tissues beyond the injection track by 2 weeks (**Fig. 9**), and had largely dispersed from the site of administration by 4 to 6 weeks. There was only minimal cell migration from the injured SDFT to adjacent sites. The tendons treated with the tendon-derived cells also had significantly increased DNA content within the lesion site during the first 2 weeks after the injection, reflecting increased cellularity. This difference was lost at later time points.

To date, only 2 cases of clinical tendonitis have been treated with tendon-derived progenitor cells (**Fig. 10**) (Dr Jennifer Barrett, personal communication, 2011). Both horses returned to performance, but 1 tendon injury recurred after 18 months.

Safety

In the studies completed to date, tendon-derived cells have been isolated from the hind limb lateral digital extensor (LDE) tendons of 8 research horses using an approach more commonly used to treat stringhalt. There were no immediate complications associated with intratendinous stem cells injections after the LDE tenectomy in the donor horses; however, the longer-term consequences of LDE tenectomy on subsequent athletic performance are not known.

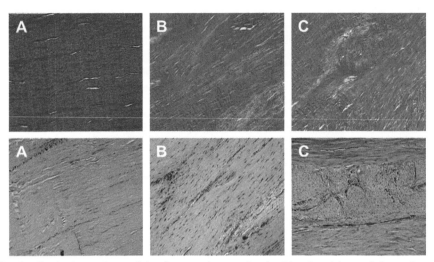

Fig. 8. Histologic sections of healing tendons stained with picrosirius red for collagen content (*upper row*) and with toluidine blue for proteoglycan content (*lower row*). (A) Normal tendon, (B) injured tendons 4 months after treatment with tendon-derived progenitor cells, and (C) injured tendons 4 months after treatment with saline injections. Fiber alignment is improved in the cell-treated lesion (comparing [B] and [C] in both rows). Collagen stains more intensively, and proteoglycan staining is less intense in the cell-treated sections (original magnification ×25).

At this time, the results from the in vivo collagenase model study have not shown a significant enough improvement in tendon healing over other MSC sources to justify the invasiveness of an LDE tenectomy to harvest the cells. However, the morphometric analyses of matrix organization and biomechanical testing of tendon specimens from this study are still ongoing, and significant beneficial effects of tendon-derived progenitor cell administration may yet be identified.

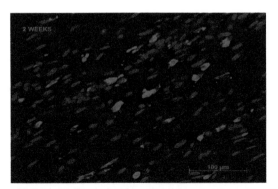

Fig. 9. Distribution of DiI-stained (*red*) tendon-derived progenitor cells after intratendinous injection. Two weeks after injection, the cells are distributed longitudinally within the healing tendon lesion and are aligned with the native tendon cells (stained blue with DAPI, original magnification ×100).

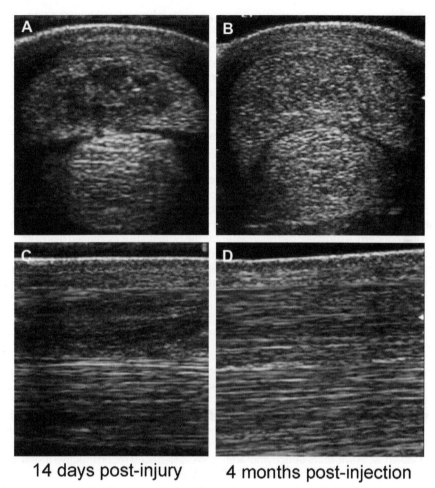

14 days post-injury   4 months post-injection

Fig. 10. Transverse (*A, B*) and longitudinal (*C, D*) ultrasonographic images of a large SDFT core lesion 14 days after injury (*A, C*) and 4 months after intralesional injection of tendon-derived stem cells. The echogenicity of the lesion has improved noticeably over this time. (*Courtesy of* Dr Jennifer Barrett, Marion duPont Scott Equine Medical Center, Virginia-Maryland Regional College of Veterinary Medicine, Leesburg, VA.)

SUMMARY

The potential for stem cells to improve or cure tendon and ligament injuries is still being investigated. There is still a need to understand the mechanisms of cell lineage commitment and the principles of tendon differentiation. Studies of both ESCs and adult stem cells will be required to advance the scientific and therapeutic potential of regenerative medicine most efficiently. Several questions need to be answered to identify the optimal cell type and dose to be identified for each clinical condition. ESCs have the greatest potential for regenerative therapy for tendons and ligaments, which have limited capacity for self-repair. However, it is clear that existing equine ESC-like cells are not yet fully characterized, and current markers used to characterize pluripotency in equine cells are inadequate. The development of iPS cells represents a possible alternative yet to be intensively investigated before its applicability is known in clinical scenarios.[57]

Adult stem cells from bone marrow have so far attracted most of the scientific attention, and both experimental data and clinical experience have suggested a positive therapeutic effect. Most importantly, MSC implantation does not result in significant deleterious effects, either from the implantation process itself or from the formation of different normal or abnormal tissues within the implantation site.[23] The work performed in natural disease in the horse provides more relevant efficacy and safety data to pave the way for their use for treating tendon and ligament injuries in other species, including man.

At present, most cell therapeutic techniques for horses have been autologous in nature. However, an allogenic source would provide an off-the-shelf product, which could then be given at an optimum time in the disease process rather than one governed by isolation and culture times. This would also potentially make the product cheaper. In addition, the product could be standardized more easily, although maintaining this standard throughout the multiple population doublings necessary to supply sufficient cells is a concern. Allogeneic cell sources entail the potential for increased risk of immunologic reaction, although MSCs are immunoprivileged and additionally suppress the immune response. In addition, allogenic cells could be a possible source of disease transmission, so further quality control and regulatory issues would need to be established.

REFERENCES

1. Butler DL, Juncosa-Melvin N, Boivin GP, et al. Functional tissue engineering for tendon repair: a multidisciplinary strategy using mesenchymal stem cells, bioscaffolds, and mechanical stimulation. J Orthop Res 2008;26(1):1–9.
2. Goodman SA, May SA, Heinegard D, et al. Tenocyte response to cyclical strain and transforming growth factor beta is dependent upon age and site of origin. Biorheology 2004;41(5):613–28.
3. Caplan AI. Review: mesenchymal stem cells: cell-based reconstructive therapy in orthopedics. Tissue Eng 2005;11(7–8):1198–211.
4. Guest DJ, Smith MR, Allen WR. Equine embryonic stem-like cells and mesenchymal stromal cells have different survival rates and migration patterns following their injection into damaged superficial digital flexor tendon. Equine Vet J 2010; 42(7):636–42.
5. Bi Y, Ehirchiou D, Kilts TM, et al. Identification of tendon stem/progenitor cells and the role of the extracellular matrix in their niche. Nat Med 2007;13(10):1219–27.
6. Smith JJ, Ross MW, Smith RK. Anabolic effects of acellular bone marrow, platelet rich plasma, and serum on equine suspensory ligament fibroblasts in vitro. Vet Comp Orthop Traumatol 2006;19(1):43–7.
7. Salingcarnboriboon R, Yoshitake H, Tsuji K, et al. Establishment of tendon-derived cell lines exhibiting pluripotent mesenchymal stem cell-like property. Exp Cell Res 2003;287(2):289–300.
8. Rehman J, Traktuev D, Li J, et al. Secretion of angiogenic and antiapoptotic factors by human adipose stromal cells. Circulation 2004;109(10):1292–8.
9. Haynesworth SE, Baber MA, Caplan AI. Cytokine expression by human marrow-derived mesenchymal progenitor cells in vitro: effects of dexamethasone and IL-1 alpha. J Cell Physiol 1996;166(3):585–92.
10. Sorrell JM, Baber MA, Caplan AI. Influence of adult mesenchymal stem cells on in vitro vascular formation. Tissue Eng Part A 2009;15(7):1751–61.

11. Herrero C, Pérez-Simón JA. Immunomodulatory effect of mesenchymal stem cells. Braz J Med Biol Res 2010;43(5):425–30.

12. Ren G, Zhang L, Zhao X, et al. Mesenchymal stem cell-mediated immunosuppression occurs via concerted action of chemokines and nitric oxide. Cell Stem Cell 2008;2(2):141–50.

13. Nixon AJ, Dahlgren LA, Haupt JL, et al. Effect of adipose-derived nucleated cell fractions on tendon repair in horses with collagenase-induced tendinitis. Am J Vet Res 2008;69(7):928–37.

14. Carvalho A, Alves A, de Oliveira P, et al. Use of adipose tissue-derived mesenchymal stem cells for experimental tendinitis therapy in equines. J Equine Vet Sci 2011;31:26–34.

15. Murphy JM, Fink DJ, Hunziker EB, et al. Stem cell therapy in a caprine model of osteoarthritis. Arthritis Rheum 2003;48(12):3464–74.

16. Caplan AI. Mesenchymal stem cells. J Orthop Res 1991;9(5):641–50.

17. Fortier LA, Travis AJ. Stem cells in veterinary medicine. Stem Cell Res Ther 2011; 2(1):9.

18. Radcliffe CH, Flaminio MJ, Fortier LA. Temporal analysis of equine bone marrow aspirate during establishment of putative mesenchymal progenitor cell populations. Stem Cells Dev 2010;19(2):269–82.

19. Toupadakis CA, Wong A, Genetos DC, et al. Comparison of the osteogenic potential of equine mesenchymal stem cells from bone marrow, adipose tissue, umbilical cord blood, and umbilical cord tissue. Am J Vet Res 2010;71(10): 1237–45.

20. Im GI, Shin YW, Lee KB. Do adipose tissue-derived mesenchymal stem cells have the same osteogenic and chondrogenic potential as bone marrow-derived cells? Osteoarthritis Cartilage 2005;13(10):845–53.

21. Vidal MA, Kilroy GE, Lopez MJ, et al. Characterization of equine adipose tissue-derived stromal cells: adipogenic and osteogenic capacity and comparison with bone marrow-derived mesenchymal stromal cells. Vet Surg 2007;36(7):613–22.

22. Stewart AA, Barrett JG, Byron CR, et al. Comparison of equine tendon-, muscle-, and bone marrow-derived cells cultured on tendon matrix. Am J Vet Res 2009; 70(6):750–7.

23. Richardson LE, Dudhia J, Clegg PD, et al. Stem cells in veterinary medicine—attempts at regenerating equine tendon after injury. Trends Biotechnol 2007; 25(9):409–16.

24. Guest DJ, Smith MR, Allen WR. Monitoring the fate of autologous and allogeneic mesenchymal progenitor cells injected into the superficial digital flexor tendon of horses: preliminary study. Equine Vet J 2008;40(2):178–81.

25. Shukunami C, Takimoto A, Oro M, et al. Scleraxis positively regulates the expression of tenomodulin, a differentiation marker of tenocytes. Dev Biol 2006;298(1): 234–47.

26. Violini S, Ramelli P, Pisani LF, et al. Horse bone marrow mesenchymal stem cells express embryo stem cell markers and show the ability for tenogenic differentiation by in vitro exposure to BMP-12. BMC Cell Biol 2009;10:29.

27. Young RG, Butler DL, Weber W, et al. Use of mesenchymal stem cells in a collagen matrix for Achilles tendon repair. J Orthop Res 1998;16(4):406–13.

28. Awad HA, Butler DL, Boivin GP, et al. Autologous mesenchymal stem cell-mediated repair of tendon. Tissue Eng 1999;5(3):267–77.

29. Ouyang HW, Goh JC, Mo XM, et al. The efficacy of bone marrow stromal cell-seeded knitted PLGA fiber scaffold for Achilles tendon repair. Ann N Y Acad Sci 2002;961:126–9.

30. Ouyang HW, Goh JC, Thambyah A, et al. Knitted poly-lactide-co-glycolide scaffold loaded with bone marrow stromal cells in repair and regeneration of rabbit Achilles tendon. Tissue Eng 2003;9(3):431–9.
31. Hankemeier S, van Griensven M, Ezechieli M, et al. Tissue engineering of tendons and ligaments by human bone marrow stromal cells in a liquid fibrin matrix in immunodeficient rats: results of a histologic study. Arch Orthop Trauma Surg 2007;127(9):815–21.
32. Schnabel LV, Lynch ME, van der Meulen MC, et al. Mesenchymal stem cells and insulin-like growth factor-I gene-enhanced mesenchymal stem cells improve structural aspects of healing in equine flexor digitorum superficialis tendons. J Orthop Res 2009;27(10):1392–8.
33. Crovace A, Lacitignola L, De Siena R, et al. Cell therapy for tendon repair in horses: an experimental study. Vet Res Commun 2007;31(Suppl 1):281–3.
34. Crovace A, Lacitignola L, Rossi G, et al. Histological and immunohistochemical evaluation of autologous cultured bone marrow mesenchymal stem cells and bone marrow mononucleated cells in collagenase-induced tendinitis of equine superficial digital flexor tendon. Vet Med Int 2010;2010:250978.
35. Schramme M, Hunter S, Campbell N, et al. A surgical tendonitis model in horses: technique, clinical, ultrasonographic and histological characterisation. Vet Comp Orthop Traumatol 2010;23(4):231–9.
36. Godwin EE, Young NJ, Dudhia J, et al. Implantation of bone marrow-derived mesenchymal stem cells demonstrates improved outcome in horses with overstrain injury of the superficial digital flexor tendon. Equine Vet J, 2011 May 26. DOI:10.1111/j.2042-3306.2011.00363.x. [Epub ahead of print]. PubMed PMID: 21615465.
37. Dyson SJ. Medical management of superficial digital flexor tendonitis: a comparative study in 219 horses (1992–2000). Equine Vet J 2004;36(5):415–9.
38. O'Meara B, Bladon B, Parkin TD, et al. An investigation of the relationship between race performance and superficial digital flexor tendonitis in the Thoroughbred racehorse. Equine Vet J 2010;42(4):322–6.
39. Li X, Zhou SG, Imreh MP, et al. Horse embryonic stem cell lines from the proliferation of inner cell mass cells. Stem Cells Dev 2006;15(4):523–31.
40. Abavisani A, McKinnon A, Tecirlioglu R, et al. Maintenance of horse embryonic stem cells in different conditions. Iranian Journal of Veterinary Research 2010;11: 239–48.
41. Giudice A, Trounson A. Genetic modification of human embryonic stem cells for derivation of target cells. Cell Stem Cell 2008;2(5):422–33.
42. Nagy K, Sung HK, Zhang P, et al. Induced pluripotent stem cell lines derived from equine fibroblasts. Stem Cell Rev 2011. DOI:10.1007/s12015-011-9239-5.
43. Thomson JA, Itskovitz-Eldor J, Shapiro SS, et al. Embryonic stem cell lines derived from human blastocysts. Science 1998;282(5391):1145–7.
44. Saito S, Sawai K, Minamihashi A, et al. Derivation, maintenance, and induction of the differentiation in vitro of equine embryonic stem cells. Methods Mol Biol 2006; 329:59–79.
45. Saito S, Ugai H, Sawai K, et al. Isolation of embryonic stem-like cells from equine blastocysts and their differentiation in vitro. FEBS Lett 2002;531:389–96.
46. Guest DJ, Allen WR. Expression of cell-surface antigens and embryonic stem cell pluripotency genes in equine blastocysts. Stem Cells Dev 2007;16(5):789–96.
47. Hochereau-de Reviers MT, Perreau C. In vitro culture of embryonic disc cells from porcine blastocysts. Reprod Nutr Dev 1993;33(5):475–83.

48. Anderson GB, BonDurant RH, Goff L, et al. Development of bovine and porcine embryonic teratomas in athymic mice. Anim Reprod Sci 1996;45(3):231–40.
49. Thomson JA, Kalishman J, Golos TG, et al. Isolation of a primate embryonic stem cell line. Proc Natl Acad Sci U S A 1995;92(17):7844–8.
50. Paris DB, Stout TA. Equine embryos and embryonic stem cells: defining reliable markers of pluripotency. Theriogenology 2010;74(4):516–24.
51. Smith RK, Birch HL, Goodman S, et al. The influence of ageing and exercise on tendon growth and degeneration—hypotheses for the initiation and prevention of strain-induced tendinopathies. Comp Biochem Physiol A Mol Integr Physiol 2002; 133(4):1039–50.
52. Herthel D. Enhanced suspensory ligament healing in 100 horses by stem cells and other bone marrow components. Proc Am Assoc Equine Pract 2001;47:319.
53. Barrett JG, Stewart AA, Yates AC, et al. Tendon-derived progenitor cells can differentiate along multiple lineages. Proc 34th Ann Conf Vet Ortho Soc 2007; 34:31.
54. De Mos M, Koevoet W, Jahr H, et al. Intrinsic differentiation potential of adolescent human tendon tissue: and in vitro cell differentiation study. BMC Musculoskelet Disord 2007;8:16.
55. Jankowski R, Haluszczak C, Trucco M, et al. Flow cytometric characterization of myogenic cell populations obtained via the pre-plate technique: potential for rapid isolation of muscle-derived stem cells. Hum Gene Ther 2001;12:619–28.
56. Durgam SS, Stewart AA, Pondenis H, et al. Responses of equine tendon- and bone marrow-derived cells to monolayer expansion with FGF-2 and sequential culture with IGF-I and pulverized tendon. Am J Vet Res 2010. Accepted for publication.
57. Smith RK. 'Can you regain your youth?'—the real potential of stem cell technology. Equine Vet J 2010;42(1):2–4.

Cell-based Therapies for Equine Joint Disease

David D. Frisbie, DVM, PhD[a,b,*], Matthew C. Stewart, BVSc, MVetClinStud, PhD[c]

KEYWORDS

- Intra-articular disease • Cell-based therapy • Osteoarthritis
- Soft tissue injury • Cartilage • Resurfacing

Cell-based therapies for the treatment of equine articular disease have been reported for almost three decades, driven by the significant impact of joint disease on performance horses, the inadequate reparative capacity of articular cartilage, and the limitations of current medical and surgical options for treating established arthritis. Although most joint injuries have myriad damages that cannot be confined to basic categories, this article addresses therapy for joint disease in three main categories of articular tissue damage: (1) cartilage injury/resurfacing, (2) generalized osteoarthritis (OA), and (3) intra-articular soft tissue injury (eg, meniscal).

CARTILAGE INJURY/RESURFACING

Articular cartilage is notorious for its limited ability to undergo effective repair[1–5] in part as a consequence of the relatively hypocellular and avascular nature of the tissue. This limitation is compounded in performance horses by the extreme loading stresses that are placed on articular surfaces during high-level competition. Many strategies have been developed in an attempt to regenerate functional articular cartilage, with mixed results. In people, total joint replacement continues to be the gold standard for treatment of advanced joint disease, but several techniques have proved effective for focal

Disclosure. Dr Frisbie is a shareholder in Advanced Regenerative Technologies, 200 West Mountain Suite A, Fort Collins, CO 80521; (970) 222-9831; www.art4dvm.com.
[a] Equine Orthopaedic Research Center, Department of Clinical Sciences, College of Veterinary Medicine and Biological Sciences, Colorado State University, 300 West Drake Road, Fort Collins, CO 80523, USA
[b] Molecular, Cellular and Tissue Engineering, Department of Mechanical Engineering, School of Biomedical Engineering, Colorado State University, Fort Collins, CO, USA
[c] Department of Veterinary Clinical Medicine, College of Veterinary Medicine, University of Illinois, 1008 West Hazelwood Drive, Urbana, IL 61802, USA
* Corresponding author.
E-mail address: David.Frisbie@ColoState.EDU

Vet Clin Equine 27 (2011) 335–349
doi:10.1016/j.cveq.2011.06.005

cartilage lesion repair. Apart from the direct relevance of cartilage repair for equine athletes, the horse has served as an excellent experimental model for cartilage repair investigations.

Grafting Techniques

Early experimental studies assessed the value of periosteal graft onlays[6,7] and sternal autografts[8,9] for resurfacing the distal articular surface of the equine radial carpal bone. Although the short-term results with sternal cartilage grafting were promising,[8] neither technique proved clinically viable. Osteochondral grafting (OCG) was demonstrated as technically feasible in horses,[10,11] and OCG mosaic arthroplasty has been used successfully in several cases of focal cystic lesions of the distal femoral condyles, distal metacarpal and metatarsal bones, and talus.[12,13] OCG was of only of marginal benefit for third carpal bone lesions, due to synovial hyperplasia at the graft site and the excessive loads experienced by the dorsal margins of the carpal bones.[14,15]

OCG mosaic arthroplasty carries limitations: available donor sites are limited, graft collection entails an additional surgical procedure and creates donor site morbidity, and successful outcomes are highly dependent on technical proficiency in seating the grafts securely and restoring a congruent articular surface.[10] OCGs represent an alternative option for mosaic arthroplasty and, despite documented concerns related to immunogenicity and detrimental host reactions,[16] the long-term results in people are encouraging.[17,18] Little assessment of equine osteochondral allograft utility has been performed, but preliminary work by Pearce and colleagues[11] suggest that allografting is a feasible approach for focal articular cartilage repair, provided suitable tissue collection and storage protocols and facilities are established.

Microfracture

In 1999, the first report of equine subchondral bone microfracture was published,[19] after the development of this technique by Blevins and colleagues[20] and Steadman and colleagues.[20,21] Microfracture provides access for chondrogenic progenitor cells in the subchondral bone marrow compartment into the base of the cartilage defect.[22,23] A study by Frisbie and colleagues demonstrated a clear benefit of microfracture for equine cartilage resurfacing compared to standard debridement alone.[19] Twelve months after surgery, microfractured defects had significantly more repair tissue infill (74%) than the control defects (45%), and the percentage of type II collagen in treated defects was higher than in the control defects.

Subsequent studies have demonstrated that cartilage repair after microfracture is dependent in part on complete removal of the calcified cartilage layer directly above the subchondral bone plate.[24] Cartilage repair following microfracture can also be improved by filling the defect with a fibrin gel loaded with insulin-like growth factor 1 (IGF-1),[25] through intra-articular gene therapy delivery of IGF-1 and interleukin receptor antagonist,[26] or by filling the cartilage defect with bone marrow concentrate gelled by addition of thrombin.[27] This last technique is notable in that, although the application of the bone marrow concentrate requires gas insufflation of the joint space, the biologic supplement is readily collected and can be prepared at the time of the primary surgery.

Chondrocyte-based Strategies

Implantation of ex vivo expanded articular chondrocyte implantation (ACI) is a commonly performed procedure in people with focal cartilage defects and carries a favorable prognosis for improvement in clinical signs.[28–30] There are problems associated with the need for two procedures, donor site morbidity, chondrocyte phenotypic instability, and scaffold/patch delamination, but ACI is particularly applicable for larger (>4 cm^2) femoral condylar lesions in young adults with minimal degenerative changes in the affected joint.[31] ACI has been shown effective for both short-term and long-term repair of large partial-thickness and full-thickness articular cartilage defects in horses[32,33]; however, the complexity of the initial cartilage collection, ex vivo expansion, and surgical reimplantation makes this approach unfeasible for the majority of equine surgical practices. A 2009 study by Frisbie and colleagues[19] also assessed the clinical utility of autologous cartilage fragment implantation for cartilage defect repair. This approach was as effective as ACI in stimulating cartilage repair and has the major advantage that it can be applied during a single surgical procedure in an appropriately equipped facility. Access to the proprietary membrane and staples still remains a limitation for routine equine practice.

Over the past two decades, a number of studies have been carried out in equine models to assess the value of chondrocyte transplantation for the repair of articular cartilage defects. Early studies confirmed that allogeneic chondrocyte transplantation in a fibrin matrix resulted in significantly improved outcomes,[34] although repair using collagen-based scaffolds was not successful.[35] In a subsequent study, transplanted chondrocytes were delivered in fibrin gels supplemented with IGF-1 protein.[36] After 8 months, the histologic appearance of the cartilage defect treated with IGF-1was substantially improved over that of the controls; however, biochemical differences of the repair tissues were less notable and biomechanical testing of the repaired tissue showed no effect of IGF-1 supplementation.[37] Using gene therapy approaches, articular chondrocytes were genetically modified to express high levels of IGF-1[38] or bone morphogenetic protein (BMP) 7,[39] using adenoviral vectors. Both these secreted factors are known to support the differentiated chondrocytic phenotype and stimulate cartilage matrix synthesis. In both studies, overexpression of IGF-1 or BMP7 stimulated impressive early repair within the cartilage defects but the longer-term results were less significant. In light of the sophisticated ex vivo manipulation of chondrocytes that these techniques entail, the specialized facilities required for chondrocyte:fibrin matrix implantation, the attendant costs associated with these procedures, and the lack of compelling outcome data from clinical cases to date, these methods have not gained significant clinical usage in equine medicine and are likely to remain restricted to highly specialized referral practices.

Stem Cell–based Strategies

Given their ability to undergo chondrogenic differentiation, much of the cartilage resurfacing research effort in recent years has focused on the use of mesenchymal stem cells (MSCs). Experimental studies using distal femoral condylar defect models in laboratory animal models (for examples, see Refs.[40–44]) have generally shown an improved reparative response with MSC delivery to the defect site, but it is difficult to determine the clinical relevance of these outcomes to cartilage repair in larger and more mobile species, such as the horse.

A few clinical outcomes in people have been reported by Wakitani and colleagues[45] after MSC implantation into patellofemoral cartilage lesions. In the first report, bone marrow aspirates were collected from the iliac crest of 3 patients 3 weeks before the cartilage repair procedure and bone marrow MSCs were expanded in monolayer culture using autologous serum. The ex vivo expanded bone marrow MSCs were resuspended in a collagen solution, seeded onto a collagen sheet, implanted in the cartilage defect, and covered with a periosteal or synovial flap in a procedure somewhat analogous to ACI. All 3 patients showed modest clinical improvement at the 6-month reassessment and the improvements were sustained for 17 to 27 months after implantation, despite an MRI assessment of 1 patient 12 months after the procedure showing incomplete repair of the lesion and biopsy of another patient 11 months after MSC administration demonstrating a predominantly fibrocartilaginous repair. In the second report, the outcomes of 12 femoral condylar lesions treated with MSCs in collagen gel were compared with repair in 12 lesions filled with the collagen gel alone.[46] The patients enrolled in this study were all undergoing high tibial osteotomies for knee arthritis. The quality of the repair response was monitored via follow-up arthroscopic assessments and needle biopsies of the repair tissue, ranging from 28 to 95 weeks after the initial repair. Although there were no significant clinical differences between the treatment and control groups, the histologic and arthroscopic appearance of the MSC-treated defects were improved. Although these clinical studies are somewhat anecdotal and the clinical improvements that followed MSC implantation were modest at best, these reports validate the feasibility of MSC implantation in human and, by extension, veterinary patients.

To date, the published literature on articular cartilage repair in using MSCs in the horse is limited. A technique that utilizes a fibrin scaffold to retain MSCs within cartilage defects has been developed; however this strategy necessitates that autologous MSCs are prepared before arthroscopy. This approach has the disadvantage of leaving the need for MSCs uncertain until diagnostic arthroscopy is performed and a suitable lesion identified. Thus, if an appropriate lesion is not identified during arthroscopic evaluation, this approach is not the best use of resources. Arthroscopic implantation of MSC scaffolds also requires specialized equipment, in particular, gas insufflation of the joint cavity. A controlled experimental study using surgically created 15-mm cartilage defects in the lateral trochlear ridge of the distal femur did not demonstrate long-term benefits to cartilage repair after MSC implantation.[47]

Independent of their ability to participate in and/or influence tissue repair, MSCs have been used experimentally for local gene delivery (reviewed by Gafni and colleageus[48]). Delivery of MSCs transduced with adenoviral vectors expressing BMP ligands improved the quality of cartilage repair in both rat and rabbit distal femoral defect models.[49,50] Although it might be expected that the overexpressed genes would dominate the biologic responses to transgene-activated MSCs, a study performed in the rat distal femur by Park and colleagues[50] demonstrated marked effects derived from the MSC source. In this study, adipose-derived MSCs overexpressing BMP2 were far less capable of generating a cartilage-like repair tissue than BMP2 transduced perichondrial-derived or bone marrow–derived MSCs. In both these studies, the control defects treated with naïve MSCs were filled with fibrous and fibrocartilaginous tissues only, suggesting that the chondrogenic capacity of MSCs alone was inadequate for effective repair.

Another promising strategy involves injecting MSCs directly into the joint space, without the use of a scaffold, 30 days after diagnostic arthroscopy, thus avoiding MSC collection and preparation before ascertaining the need for this therapy. The timing of this treatment application was based on return to athletic use in a group of clinically treated horses that were followed for an average of 21 months. Delayed MSC injection resulted in improved repair of 1-cm^2 medial femoral condylar defects compared to subchondral bone microfracture alone in a long-term strenuous exercise in vivo model. The control joints were treated with hyaluronan (HA), whereas the contralateral joint received HA and 2×10^6 MSCs. Both treatments were injected directly into the joint space 30 days after lesion creation. After a year of strenuous exercise, some softening of the microfracture alone (HA only) repair tissue was noted but the repair tissue in the MSC-treated joint remained firm compared with a 6-month time point.[51] Furthermore, the degree of aggrecan staining was improved in the MSC-treated repair tissue when compared with microfracture alone at the 12-month time point. Based on this work, along with the findings of Lee and colleagues,[52] who also administered MSCs into the joint space in a porcine model, it seems that direct intra-articular administration of MSCs is a more straightforward therapy and may have long-term advantages compared with delivering the cells directly to the defect site within a fibrin scaffold.

Bioscaffold-based Strategies

In recent years, articular cartilage regeneration has become something of a holy grail for the bioengineering community. With the development of increasingly sophisticated tissue engineering approaches, which include biocompatible and resorbable polymeric, hydrogel, and bioceramic scaffold materials,[40,53,54] biphasic composites that recapitulate the appropriate niches for chondrogenic and/or osteogenic differentiation of MSCs,[55–57] self-assembling peptide hydrogels,[58] and scaffolds that deliver morphogenetic factors in a controlled manner,[59,60] extrinsic cell delivery to cartilage defects could well become unnecessary. In several studies (referred to previously), the acellular bioscaffolds performed as effectively as cell-seeded scaffolds for articular cartilage regeneration. With ongoing research and development, bioscaffolds might be capable of recruiting appropriate progenitor cells and providing the requisite physical and soluble cues to stimulate optimal repair/regeneration. Self-evidently, this strategy is dependent on a competent reparative cell population available in the host/patient for recruitment.

GENERALIZED OSTEOARTHRITIS

The treatment of OA, whether by cell-based therapies or more conventional approaches, is considerably more challenging than the repair of focal cartilage defects. In OA joints, articular cartilage pathology is often diffuse and involves both articulating surfaces; other articular and periarticular tissues (synovial membrane, joint capsule, ligaments, menisci, and subchondral bone) are also involved in the pathologic basis of the disease (**Fig. 1**A). In horses, articular margins (for example, the dorsal margins of the radial and third carpal bones and the dorso-proximal rim of the first phalanx) are commonly involved, as opposed to the discreet, focal cartilage lesions that are amenable to resurfacing procedures. With specific regard to cell-based therapies, OA joints are variably inflammatory environments, and chondrocytes within OA joints are phenotypically and biosynthetically dysfunctional by several criteria (see **Fig. 1**B, C).[61–63] Furthermore, there is some evidence that stem cells from arthritic patients are dysfunctional compared with their normal counterparts,[64] although this finding has not been consistently reported.[65,66]

As shown by Koelling and colleagues,[23] a population of chondrogenic precursor cells resides in the subchondral bone compartment and migrates into chondral repair tissue in advanced OA. The synovial fluid for OA joints contains a range of cell-attractant chemokines, most notably CXCL10,[67] and subchondral mesenchymal progenitor cells are responsive to these chemotactic signals. Furthermore, OA articular chondrocytes secrete morphogenetic factors that stimulate chondrogenic differentiation of MSCs with phenotypic characteristics of articular, as opposed to endochondral, chondrocyte populations.[68] These observations provide a molecular rationale for the clinical efficacy of microfracture techniques but, in an untreated OA joint environment, recruitment of subchondral chondroprogenitor cells can only occur after arthritic pathology has reached an advanced state and the calcified cartilage tidemark has been penetrated. Intrinsic cellular responses are inadequate to reverse

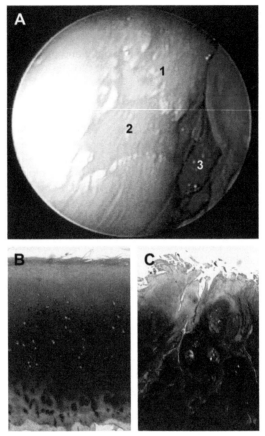

Fig. 1. Pathologic changes in equine OA. As seen in the arthroscopic view (A), OA involves fibrillation and fissuring of articular cartilage (1); complete cartilage loss, with associated alterations to the subchondral bone (2); and both hyperplasia and hyperemia of the synovial membrane (3). Comparison of the histologic appearance of intact (B) and advanced OA (C) cartilage demonstrates the profound changes that occur in arthritic cartilage (sections stained with toluidine blue). The intact cartilage section (B) has mild surface fibrillation, whereas the advanced OA section (C) shows deep fissure formation, marked surface irregularity and proteoglycan loss (pale regions), reduced cell density, and prominent chondrocyte clustering. Clinically effective arthritis therapy needs to address the pathologic changes in multiple tissues and the often advanced degenerative changes present in the articular cartilage itself.

or arrest disease progression by this stage. This has led to the development of several strategies to apply the regenerative and reparative activities of MSCs more effectively in OA joints.

MSCs are capable of adhering to articular cartilage surfaces in the absence of other substrates,[69,70] but several studies using cell-labeling techniques have shown that, after intra-articular injection, MSCs preferentially localize to articular soft tissue structures with little or no adherence of injected cells to the cartilage surface[70–73] and little or no retention within cartilage defects.[52,70,71] In light of these results, any beneficial effects of intra-articularly administered MSCs on articular cartilage are likely mediated by soluble factors or by primary effects on other articular tissues. In inflammatory arthritic conditions, MSCs inhibit activation of T lymphocytes and secretion of inflammatory cytokines while concurrently stimulating secretion of anti-inflammatory interleukins[74,75] and reducing consequent articular tissue damage.[76] Furthermore, in vitro studies indicate that, under inflammatory conditions, MSCs effectively antagonize MMP activity by secreting tissue inhibitors of metalloproteinases.[77] These MSC-mediated activities could be clinically beneficial in OA joints and support chondrocyte metabolism in the face of arthritic disease.

Several studies have demonstrated beneficial responses after intra-articular MSC administration. In a rabbit anterior cruciate ligament (ACL) transection model, Grigolo and colleagues[78] applied autologous bone marrow MSCs impregnated into an esterified hyaluronate mesh (Hyaff-11) onto the femoral condylar surfaces, 8 weeks after stifle joint destabilization. The contralateral control joints received acellular hyaluronate scaffolds. Histologic, histomorphometric, and immunohistological evaluations were performed 3 and 6 months after ACL transection and demonstrated significant improvements in the status of the MSC-treated articular cartilage. Using a similar lapine model, Toghraie and colleagues[79] injected 1 million allogeneic MSCs derived from infrapatellar fat pad 12 weeks after joint destabilization. The effects of MSC administration were assessed after a further 8 weeks. Intra-articular MSC injection reduced cartilage degeneration, osteophyte formation, and subchondral bone sclerosis. Accepting that the rabbit stifle joint is a forgiving model for articular cartilage repair and arthritis progression, MSC administration was performed after the establishment of arthritic pathology in both studies, and the serial analyses of cartilage histology (and radiologic assessments by Toghraie and colleagues[79]) suggest that MSC administration reversed some of the pathologic changes in this model, as opposed to merely slowing the progression of arthritis. A single human case study also suggests that intra-articularly administered MSCs can restore articular cartilage volume, as assessed by MRI, and improve clinical signs of arthritic disease for several months after administration.[80]

The effect of intra-articular MSC administration was assessed in a more challenging model by Murphy and colleagues.[73] In this study, caprine femorotibial joints were destabilized by transecting the ACL and excising the medial meniscus. Postoperatively, the goats were exercised to induce OA. Autologous bone marrow MSCs were administered intra-articularly 6 weeks after joint destabilization. The effects of treatment were assessed 6 and 20 weeks after the intra-articular injections. Indices of articular cartilage degeneration and subchondral sclerosis were reduced in the MSC-treated joints at the 6-week assessment, but this protective effect was not as evident at 20 weeks. The remarkable finding in this study was the impressive and rapid regeneration of a neomeniscus-like pannus in 7 of the 9 cell-treated joints. The investigators concluded that the decrease in OA seen in the MSC-treated joints was largely secondary to the stabilizing and chondroprotective effects of the meniscal regenerate, because the 2 MSC-treated cases that did not generate a neomeniscus exhibited early cartilage degeneration, as seen in the control joints. The experimental method for inducing OA did not lend itself, however, to determining if the MSCs also had a direct effect on articular cartilage and/or progression of OA.

A subsequent equine study was performed in an established carpal osteochondral fragment model, in which bone and cartilage debris induces OA but joint destabilization is minimal.[81] The goal of the study was twofold: first, to evaluate the effects of bone marrow–derived, culture-expanded MSCs and adipose-derived stromal vascular cell fraction (ADSVF) on acute OA, and second, to compare the efficacies of the 2 cell-based treatment modalities. The results of this study indicated significant improvement in synovial fluid protaglandin E_2 levels in response to treatment with bone marrow–derived cells, although significant differences were not demonstrated in other key parameters (clinical lameness, radiographic, histologic, and biochemical assessments). The study also demonstrated an increase in synovial fluid tumor necrosis factor α concentrations in response to adipose-derived cell administration, which could be interpreted in a negative light. The conclusion of this equine study was that nominal improvement in clinical signs and disease-modifying effects were seen with bone marrow–derived stem cells. Furthermore, ADSVF administration up-regulated synovial fluid concentrations of proinflammatory cytokines. This stable acute OA model raises questions regarding the utility of intra-articular MSC injections for the treatment of equine OA that involves significant articular cartilage damage. These issues need to be critically assessed through further research and follow-up clinical results.

INTRA-ARTICULAR SOFT TISSUE INJURY

Accepting concerns regarding the efficacy of MSC therapy for articular cartilage injury, several lines of evidence indicate that stem cell therapy is beneficial for the treatment of meniscal injury. As discussed previously, MSCs bind to menisci after intra-articular administration[71,73] and bone marrow MSCs have been used successfully to colonize acellular meniscal allografts, synthesize a viable extracellular matrix, and regenerate a functional meniscal transplant in rat models.[82–84] Similar results were reported by Walsh and colleagues[85] in a rabbit partial meniscectomy model. MSC-seeded collagen scaffolds stimulated a fibrocartilaginous repair of the meniscal defect, although some degenerative changes developed despite meniscal repair in this study. In a challenging porcine model, where a radial tear was created in the avascular zone of the meniscus, the addition of MSCs to the fibrin glue and suture repair significantly improved outcomes but did not effect successful healing in all subjects.[86] Percutaneous administration of 45 million bone marrow MSCs into a human patient's femorotibial joint increased medial meniscal volume over a 3-month interval, as assessed by MRI,[87] although this patient also received intra-articular marrow aspirate, hyaluronan, and pulsed ultrasound therapy for 3 weeks after the injection. The meniscal changes were associated with noticeable improvements in clinical signs related to knee pain. Most compellingly, the study by Murphy and colleagues[73] (discussed previously) demonstrated the capacity of intra-articularly delivered MSCs to stimulate rapid functional meniscal regeneration.

In attempts to replicate the beneficial results seen by Murphy and colleagues,[73] researchers at Colorado State University have been treating various clinical cases of joint disease with arthroscopically confirmed soft tissue injury using a combination of HA and MSCs.[88] These efforts have been particularly focused on those cases diagnosed with meniscal injury. A 6-month follow-up pilot project involving 15 cases showed promising results and led the investigators to expand the study into a multicenter trial. The results of this prospective multicenter trail were also promising.[89] To date, 39 cases have been treated with intra-articular administration of autologous bone marrow–derived MSCs, with a mean follow-up period of 21 months. Patients selected for this trial were nonresponsive to routine treatments, were moderately to severely affected, and the majority of cases had arthroscopically confirmed meniscal damage. Seventy-seven percent of patients have returned to some level of work; 36% (14/39) returned to or exceeded their prior level of work; 36% (14/39) returned to work at a lower level of performance or required additional medical treatment in the affected joint to maintain soundness; and 28% (11/39) did not achieve their former work status before follow-up.[88] Stifle injuries comprised 29 of the 39 cases, with 20 having a primary diagnosis of meniscal damage.

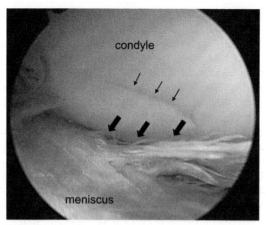

Fig. 2. Meniscal pathology. Clinical case studies by researchers at Colorado State University suggest that stifle lameness cases associated with meniscal injuries (*large black arrows*) but with little or no cartilage damage (*thin black arrows*) respond well to intra-articular MSC injections. (*Courtesy of* Santiago Gutierrez-Nibeyro, Department of Veterinary Clinical Medicine, College of Veterinary Medicine, University of Illinois.)

Differences were noted when these data were compared with published studies on meniscal damage with surgery alone.[90,91] With surgery alone, grade 3 meniscal tears had 0 and 6% success rates for return to work compared with the current study where MSC injection and surgery resulted in a 60% return to work. Intra-articular treatment with autologous cells had an 8% incidence of acute inflammation, or flare, which, given the concurrent administration of HA (12% flare incidence reported), would be an expected, or lower than expected, outcome. At this stage, it seems that for clinical cases of equine joint disease with confirmed soft tissue involvement, especially more severe cases, administration of autogenous bone marrow–derived stem cells may improve a horse's ability to return to work over surgery alone (**Fig. 2**). The next logical step is a blinded, placebo-controlled clinical trial. This is unlikely because of difficulties regarding owner compliance for such a study design; however, a positive-control clinical trial may be feasible and could shed more light on the most useful treatment applications for cell-based therapies.

In conclusion, using endogenous cells accessed through subchondral bone microfracture seems to be the current state of the art for equine cartilage resurfacing. It seems that the outcome of this technique can be significantly augmented with timely administration of MSCs into the joint space. There is evidence that MSCs are not effective in all cases of OA but there is not yet enough information to draw definitive conclusions regarding specific types of OA and specific tissue lesions present in OA joints. Finally, there is evidence that augmenting surgery with MSC administration improves the return to work of horses suffering from severe meniscal injury. Accepting that the use of MSCs for the treatment of joint injury is an evolving therapy, it seems that they will provide benefit to equine patients, but there is much to learn.

REFERENCES

1. Vachon A, Bramlage LR, Gabel AA, et al. Evaluation of the repair process of cartilage defects of the equine third carpal bone with and without subchondral bone perforation. Am J Vet Res 1986;47(12):2637–45.

2. Hurtig MB, Fretz PB, Doige CE, et al. Effects of lesion size and location on equine articular cartilage repair. Can J Vet Res 1988;52(1):137–46.

3. Hanie EA, Sullins KE, Powers BE, et al. Healing of full-thickness cartilage compared with full-thickness cartilage and subchondral bone defects in the equine third carpal bone. Equine Vet J 1992;24(5):382–6.

4. Strauss EJ, Goodrich LR, Chen CT, et al. Biochemical and biomechanical properties of lesion and adjacent articular cartilage after chondral defect repair in an equine model. Am J Sports Med 2005;33(11):1647–53.

5. White LM, Sussman MS, Hurtig M, et al. Cartilage T2 assessment: Differentiation of normal hyaline cartilage and reparative tissue after arthroscopic cartilage repair in equine subjects. Radiology 2006;241(2):407–14.

6. Vachon AM, McIlwraith CW, Trotter GW, et al. Morphologic study of repair of induced osteochondral defects of the distal portion of the radial carpal bone in horses by use of glued periosteal autografts. Am J Vet Res 1991;52(2):317–27.

7. Vachon AM, McIlwraith CW, Keeley FW. Biochemical study of repair of induced osteochondral defects of the distal portion of the radial carpal bone in horses by use of periosteal autografts. Am J Vet Res 1991;52(2):328–32.

8. Vachon AM, McIlwraith CW, Powers BE, et al. Morphologic and biochemical study of sternal cartilage autografts for resurfacing induced osteochondral defects in horses. Am J Vet Res 1992;53(6):1038–47.

9. Howard RD, McIlwraith CW, Trotter GW, et al. Long-term fate and effects of exercise on sternal cartilage autografts used for repair of large osteochondral defects in horses. Am J Vet Res 1994;55(8):1158–67.

10. Desjardins MR, Hurtig MB, Palmer NC. Incorporation of fresh and cryopreserved bone in osteochondral autografts in the horse. Vet Surg 1991;20(6):446–52.

11. Pearce SG, Hurtig MB, Boure LP, et al. Cylindrical press-fit osteochondral allografts for resurfacing the equine metatarsophalangeal joint. Vet Surg 2003;32(3):220–30.

12. Bodo G, Hangody L, Modis L, et al. Autologous osteochondral grafting (mosaic arthroplasty) for treatment of subchondral cystic lesions in the equine stifle and fetlock joints. Vet Surg 2004;33(6):588–96.

13. Janicek JC, Cook JL, Wilson DA, et al. Multiple osteochondral autografts for treatment of a medial trochlear ridge subchondral cystic lesion in the equine tarsus. Vet Surg 2010;39(1):95–100.

14. Hurtig MB. Experimental use of small osteochondral grafts for resurfacing the equine third carpal bone. Equine Vet J Suppl 1988;6:23–7.

15. Hurtig M, Pearce S, Warren S, et al. Arthroscopic mosaic arthroplasty in the equine third carpal bone. Vet Surg 2001;30(3):228–39.

16. Stevenson S, Dannucci GA, Sharkey NA, et al. The fate of articular cartilage after transplantation of fresh and cryopreserved tissue-antigen-matched and mismatched osteochondral allografts in dogs. J Bone Joint Surg Am 1989;71(9):1297–307.

17. Hennig A, Abate J. Osteochondral allografts in the treatment of articular cartilage injuries of the knee. Sports Med Arthrosc 2007;15(3):126–32.

18. Williams SK, Amiel D, Ball ST, et al. Analysis of cartilage tissue on a cellular level in fresh osteochondral allograft retrievals. Am J Sports Med 2007;35(12):2022–32.

19. Frisbie DD, Trotter GW, Powers BE, et al. Arthroscopic subchondral bone plate microfracture technique augments healing of large chondral defects in the radial carpal bone and medical femoral condyle of horses. Vet Surg 1999;28(4):242–55.

20. Blevins FT, Steadman JR, Rodrigo JJ, et al. Treatment of articular cartilage defects in athletes: an analysis of functional outcome and lesion appearance. Orthopedics 1998;21(7):761–7.

21. Steadman JR, Rodkey WG, Briggs KK. Microfracture to treat full-thickness chondral defects: surgical technique, rehabilitation, and outcomes. J Knee Surg 2002; 15(3):170–6.

22. Kold SE, Hickman J. An experimental study of the healing process of equine chondral and osteochondral defects. Equine Vet J 1986;18(1):18–24.

23. Koelling S, Kruegel J, Irmer M, et al. Migratory chondrogenic progenitor cells from repair tissue during the later stages of human osteoarthritis. Cell Stem Cell 2009;4(4):324–35.

24. Frisbie DD, Morisset S, Ho CP, et al. Effects of calcified cartilage on healing of chondral defects treated with microfracture in horses. Am J Sports Med 2006; 34(11):1824–30.

25. Nixon AJ, Fortier LA, Williams J, et al. Enhanced repair of extensive articular defects by insulin-like growth factor-I-laden fibrin composites. J Orthop Res 1999;17(4):475–87.

26. Morisset S, Frisbie DD, Robbins PD, et al. IL-1ra/IGF-1 gene therapy modulates repair of microfractured chondral defects. Clin Orthop Relat Res 2007;462:221–8.

27. Fortier LA, Potter HG, Rickey EJ, et al. Concentrated bone marrow aspirate improves full-thickness cartilage repair compared with microfracture in the equine model. J Bone Joint Surg Am 2010;92(10):1927–37.

28. Brittberg M, Lindahl A, Nilsson A, et al. Treatment of deep cartilage defects in the knee with autologous chondrocyte transplantation. N Engl J Med 1994;331(14): 889–95.

29. Mandelbaum B, Browne JE, Fu F, et al. Treatment outcomes of autologous chondrocyte implantation for full-thickness articular cartilage defects of the trochlea. Am J Sports Med 2007;35(6):915–21.

30. Micheli LJ, Browne JE, Erggelet C, et al. Autologous chondrocyte implantation of the knee: multicenter experience and minimum 3-year follow-up. Clin J Sport Med 2001;11(4):223–8.

31. Harris JD, Siston RA, Pan X, et al. Autologous chondrocyte implantation: A systematic review. J Bone Joint Surg Am 2010;92(12):2220–33.

32. Frisbie DD, Lu Y, Kawcak CE, et al. In vivo evaluation of autologous cartilage fragment-loaded scaffold implanted into equine articular defects and compared with autologous chondrocyte implantation. Am J Sports Med 2009;37(Suppl 1): 71S–80S.

33. Nixon AJ, Begum L, Mohammed HO, et al. Autologous chondrocyte implantation drives early chondrogenesis and organized repair in extensive full- and partial-thickness cartilage defects in an equine model. J Orthop Res 2011;29(7): 1121–30.

34. Hendrickson DA, Nixon AJ, Grande DA, et al. Chondrocyte-fibrin matrix transplants for resurfacing extensive articular cartilage defects. J Orthop Res 1994; 12(4):485–97.

35. Sams AE, Nixon AJ. Chondrocyte-laden collagen scaffolds for resurfacing extensive articular cartilage defects. Osteoarthritis Cartilage 1995;3(1):47–59.

36. Fortier LA, Lust G, Mohammed HO, et al. Insulin-like growth factor-I enhances cell-based articular cartilage repair. J Bone Joint Surg Br 2002;84(2):276–88.

37. Gratz KR, Wong VW, Chen AC, et al. Biomechanical assessment of tissue retrieved after in vivo cartilage defect repair: tensile modulus of repair tissue and integration with host cartilage. J Biomech 2006;39(1):138–46.

38. Goodrich LR, Hidaka C, Robbins PD, et al. Genetic modification of chondrocytes with insulin-like growth factor-1 enhances cartilage healing in an equine model. J Bone Joint Surg Br 2007;89(5):672–85.

39. Hidaka C, Goodrich LR, Chen C-T, et al. Acceleration of cartilage repair by genetically modified chondrocytes over expressing bone morphogenetic protein-7. J Orthop Res 2003;21(4):573–83.

40. Guo X, Wang C, Zhang Y, et al. Repair of large articular cartilage defects with implants of autologous mesenchymal stem cells seeded into β-tricalcium phosphate in a sheep model. Tissue Eng 2004;10(11–12):1818–29.

41. Guo X, Zheng Q, Yang S, et al. Repair of full-thickness articular cartilage defects by cultured mesenchymal stem cells transfected with the transforming growth factor β1 gene. Biomed Mater 2006;1(4):206–15.

42. Jung M, Kaszap B, Redöhl A, et al. Enhanced early tissue regeneration after matrix-assisted autologous mesenchymal stem cell transplantation in full thickness chondral defects in a minipig model. Cell Transplant 2009;18(8): 923–32.

43. Shao XX, Hutmacher DW, Ho ST, et al. Evaluation of a hybrid scaffold/cell construct in repair of high-load-bearing osteochondral defects in rabbits. Biomaterials 2006;27(7):1071–80.

44. Wakitani S, Goto T, Pineda SJ, et al. Mesenchymal cell-based repair of large, full-thickness defects of articular cartilage. J Bone Joint Surg Am 1994;76(4): 579–92.

45. Wakitani S, Nawata M, Tensho K, et al. Repair of articular cartilage defects in the patello-femoral joint with autologous bone marrow mesenchymal cell transplantation: three case reports involving nine defects in five knees. J Tissue Eng Regen Med 2007;1(1):74–9.

46. Wakitani S, Imoto K, Yamamoto T, et al. Human autologous culture expanded bone marrow mesenchymal cell transplantation for repair of cartilage defects in osteoarthritic knees. Osteoarthritis Cartilage 2002;10(3):199–206.

47. Wilke MM, Nydam DV, Nixon AJ. Enhanced early chondrogenesis in articular defects following arthroscopic mesenchymal stem cell implantation in an equine model. J Orthop Res 2007;25(7):913–25.

48. Gafni Y, Turgeman G, Liebergal M, et al. Stem cells as vehicles for orthopedic gene therapy. Gene Ther 2004;11(4):417–26.

49. Grande DA, Mason J, Light E, et al. Stem cells as platforms for delivery of genes to enhance cartilage repair. J Bone Joint Surg Am 2003;85(Suppl 2):111–6.

50. Park J, Gelse K, Frank S, et al. Transgene-activated mesenchymal stem cells for articular cartilage repair: a comparison of primary bone marrow-, perichondrium/periosteum- and fat-derived cells. J Gene Med 2006;8(1):112–25.

51. McIlwraith CW, Frisbie DD, Rodkey WG, et al. Evaluation of intraarticular mesenchymal stem cells to augment healing of microfractured chondral defects. Arthroscopy 2011, in press.

52. Lee KB, Hui JH, Song IC, et al. Injectable mesenchymal stem cell therapy for large cartilage defects-a porcine model. Stem Cells 2007;25(11):2964–71.

53. Løken S, Jakobsen RB, Årøen A, et al. Bone marrow mesenchymal stem cells in a hyaluronan scaffold for treatment of an osteochondral defect in a rabbit model. Knee Surg Sports Traumatol Arthrosc 2008;16(10):896–903.

54. Ponticiello MS, Schinagl RM, Kadiyala S, et al. Gelatin-based resorbable sponge as a carrier matrix for human mesenchymal stem cells in cartilage regeneration therapy. J Biomed Mater Res 2000;52(2):246–55.

55. Bosnakovski D, Mizuno M, Kim G, et al. Chondrogenic differentiation of bovine bone marrow mesenchymal stem cells (MSCs) in different hydrogels: Influence of collagen type II extracellular matrix on MSC chondrogenesis. Biotechnol Bioeng 2006;93(6):1152–63.

56. Nguyen LH, Kudva AK, Guckert NL, et al. Unique biomaterial compositions direct bone marrow stem cells into specific chondrocytic phenotypes corresponding to the various zones of articular cartilage. Biomaterials 2011;32(5):1327–38.
57. Sherwood JK, Riley SL, Palazzolo R, et al. A three-dimensional osteochondral composite scaffold for articular cartilage repair. Biomaterials 2002;23(24):4739–51.
58. Kisiday J, Jin M, Kurtz B, et al. Self-assembling peptide hydrogel fosters chondrocyte extracellular matrix production and cell division: Implications for cartilage tissue repair. Proc Natl Acad Sci U S A 2002;99(15):9996–10001.
59. Kopesky PW, Vanderploeg EJ, Kisiday JD, et al. Controlled delivery of transforming growth factor β1 by self-assembling peptide hydrogels induces chondrogenesis of bone marrow stromal cells and modulates Smad2/3 signaling. Tissue Eng Part A 2011;17(1–2):83–92.
60. Miller RE, Grodzinsky AJ, Vanderploeg EJ, et al. Effect of self-assembling peptide, chondrogenic factors, and bone marrow-derived stromal cells on osteochondral repair. Osteoarthritis Cartilage 2010;18(12):1608–19.
61. Aigner T, Fundel K, Saas J, et al. Large-scale gene expression profiling reveals major pathogenetic pathways of cartilage degeneration in osteoarthritis. Arthritis Rheum 2006;54(11):3533–44.
62. Yagi R, McBurney D, Laverty D, et al. Intrajoint comparisons of gene expression patterns in human osteoarthritis suggest a change in chondrocyte phenotype. J Orthop Res 2005;23(5):1128–38.
63. Sato T, Konomi K, Yamasaki S, et al. Comparative analysis of gene expression profiles in intact and damaged regions of human osteoarthritic cartilage. Arthritis Rheum 2006;54(3):808–17.
64. Murphy MJ, Dixon K, Beck S, et al. Reduced chondrogenic and adipogenic activity of mesenchymal stem cells from patients with advanced osteoarthritis. Arthritis Rheum 2002;46(3):704–13.
65. Dudics V, Kunstar A, Kovacs J, et al. Chondrogenic potential of mesenchymal stem cells from patients with rheumatoid arthritis and osteoarthritis: Measurements in a microculture system. Cells Tissues Organs 2009;189(5):307–16.
66. Scharstuhl A, Schewe B, Benz K, et al. Chondrogenic potential of human adult mesenchymal stem cells is independent of age or osteoarthritis etiology. Stem Cells 2007;25(12):3244–51.
67. Endres M, Andreas K, Kalwitzotably G, et al. Chemokine profile of synovial fluid from normal, osteoarthritis and rheumatoid arthritis patients: CCL25, CXCL10 and XCL1 recruit human subchondral mesenchymal progenitor cells. Osteoarthritis Cartilage 2010;18(11):1458–66.
68. Aung A, Gupta G, Majid G, et al. Osteoarthritic chondrocyte–secreted morphogens induce chondrogenic differentiation of human mesenchymal stem cells. Arthritis Rheum 2011;63(1):148–58.
69. Coleman CM, Curtin C, Barry FP, et al. Mesenchymal stem cells and osteoarthritis: Remedy or accomplice? Hum Gene Ther 2010;21(10):1239–50.
70. Koga H, Shimaya M, Muneta T, et al. Local adherent technique for transplanting mesenchymal stem cells as a potential treatment of cartilage defect. Arthritis Res Ther 2008;10(4):R84.
71. Agung M, Ochi M, Yanada S, et al. Mobilization of bone marrow-derived mesenchymal stem cells into the injured tissues after intraarticular injection and their contribution to tissue regeneration. Knee Surg Sports Traumatol Arthrosc 2006; 14(12):1307–14.
72. Jing XH, Yang L, Duan XJ, et al. In vivo MR imaging tracking of magnetic iron oxide nanoparticle labeled, engineered, autologous bone marrow mesenchymal

stem cells following intra-articular injection. Joint Bone Spine 2008;75(4): 432–8.

73. Murphy JM, Fink DJ, Hunziker EB, et al. Stem cell therapy in a caprine model of osteoarthritis. Arthritis Rheum 2003;48(12):3464–74.

74. González MA, González-Rey E, Rico L, et al. Treatment of experimental arthritis by inducing immune tolerance with human adipose-derived mesenchymal stem cells. Arthritis Rheum 2009;60(4):1006–19.

75. Zheng ZH, Li XY, Ding J, et al. Allogeneic mesenchymal stem cell and mesenchymal stem cell-differentiated chondrocyte suppress the responses of type II collagen-reactive T cells in rheumatoid arthritis. Rheumatology 2008; 47(1):22–30.

76. Augello A, Tasso R, Negrini SM, et al. Cell therapy using allogeneic bone marrow mesenchymal stem cells prevents tissue damage in collagen-induced arthritis. Arthritis Rheum 2007;56(4):1175–86.

77. Lozito TP, Tuan RS. Mesenchymal stem cells inhibit both endogenous and exogenous MMPs via secreted TIMPs. J Cell Physiol 2011;226(2):385–96.

78. Grigolo B, Lisignoli G, Desando G, et al. Osteoarthritis treated with mesenchymal stem cells on hyaluronan-based scaffold in rabbit. Tissue Eng Part C Methods 2009;15(4):647–58.

79. Toghraie FS, Chenari N, Gholipour MA, et al. Treatment of osteoarthritis with infrapatellar fat pad derived mesenchymal stem cells in rabbit. Knee 2011;18(2): 71–5.

80. Centeno CJ, Busse D, Kisiday J, et al. Increased knee cartilage volume in degenerative joint disease using percutaneously implanted, autologous mesenchymal stem cells. Pain Physician 2008;11(3):343–53.

81. Frisbie DD, Kisiday JD, Kawcak CE, et al. Evaluation of adipose derived stromal vascular fraction or bone marrow derived mesenchymal stem cells for treatment of osteoarthritis. J Orthop Res 2009;27(12):1675–80.

82. Izuta Y, Ochi M, Adachi N, et al. Meniscal repair using bone marrow-derived mesenchymal stem cells: experimental study using green fluorescent protein transgenic rats. Knee 2005;12(3):217–23.

83. Yamasaki T, Deie M, Shinomiya R, et al. Meniscal regeneration using tissue engineering with a scaffold derived from a rat meniscus and Mesenchymal stromal cells derived from rat bone marrow. J Biomed Mater Res A 2005;75(1): 23–30.

84. Yamasaki T, Deie M, Shinomiya R, et al. Transplantation of meniscus regenerated by tissue engineering with a scaffold derived from a rat meniscus and mesenchymal stromal cells derived from rat bone marrow. Artif Organs 2008;32(7): 519–24.

85. Walsh CJ, Goodman D, Caplan AI, et al. Meniscus regeneration in a rabbit partial meniscectomy model. Tissue Eng 1999;5(4):327–37.

86. Dutton AQ, Choong PF, Goh JC, et al. Enhancement of meniscal repair in the avascular zone using mesenchymal stem cells in a porcine model. J Bone Joint Surg Br 2010;92(1):169–75.

87. Centeno CJ, Busse D, Kisiday J, et al. Regeneration of meniscus cartilage in a knee treated with percutaneously implanted autologous mesenchymal stem cells. Med Hypotheses 2008;71(6):900–8.

88. Frisbie DD, Hague BA, Kisiday JD. Stem cells as a treatment for osteoarthritis. Proc Am Coll Vet Surg Vet Symp. 2007. p. 39–42.

89. Proceedings of the Annual Convention of the American Association of Equine Practitioners, 2009.

90. Cohen JM, Richardson DW, McKnight AL, et al. Long-term outcome in 44 horses with stifle lameness after arthroscopic exploration and debridement. Vet Surg 2009;38(4):543–51.

91. Walmsley JP, Phillips TJ, Townsend HG. Meniscal tears in horses: an evaluation of clinical signs and arthroscopic treatment of 80 cases. Equine Vet J 2003;35(4): 402–6.

Anti-Inflammatory and Immunomodulatory Activities of Stem Cells

John F. Peroni, DVM, MS[a],*, Dori L. Borjesson, DVM, PhD[b]

KEYWORDS

• Equine • Stem cell • Mesenchymal stem cell
• Regenerative medicine • Immunomodulation • Inflammation

The recent interest in equine stem cell biology and the rapid increase in experimental data highlight the growing attention that this topic has been receiving over the past few years. Within the field of stem cell biology, the relevance of immunobiology is of particular intrigue. It appears that optimal and effective stem cell therapy for equine patients will require a thorough analysis of the immune properties of stem cells as well as their response to immune mediators. The main goal of this review is to discuss the biology of adult mesenchymal stem cells (MSCs) in the context of immunology.

MSCs are pluripotent, self-renewing cells with the potential for tissue regeneration. These cells have been implicated in the repair of bone, cartilage, tendon, ligament, skeletal muscle, and cardiac muscle. Data also suggest that MSCs may be able to transdifferentiate into cells of ectodermal origin, such as neurons. MSCs, also defined as nonembryonic stem cells, can be derived from several tissues including amniotic fluid, umbilical cord (blood and matrix), bone marrow, adipose tissue, synovium, synovial fluid, and periodontal ligament. MSCs have a bimodal effect on the immune system, including an anti-inflammatory and an immune-enhancing response. MSCs regulate immune responses such as altering antibody production by B lymphocytes (B cells), promoting shifts in T-lymphocyte (T-cell) subtypes, and inducing immune tolerance to allogeneic transplants. MSCs also have the potential for gene delivery. This review explores the diverse clinical potential for MSCs and discusses MSC mechanisms for modulating the immune response, as well as the limitations and advantages of their immunomodulatory properties. Within the context of this review the authors highlight salient immunology concepts that may better guide the

Financial disclosure/Conflict of interest: The authors have nothing to disclose.
[a] Department of Large Animal Medicine, College of Veterinary Medicine, University of Georgia, H-322, Athens, GA 30602, USA
[b] Department of Pathology, Microbiology and Immunology, School of Veterinary Medicine, University of California, Davis, CA 95616, USA
* Corresponding author.
E-mail address: jperoni@uga.edu

Vet Clin Equine 27 (2011) 351–362
doi:10.1016/j.cveq.2011.06.003
0749-0739/11/$ – see front matter. Published by Elsevier Inc.

vetequine.theclinics.com

understanding of the interactions between MSCs and the various components of the immune system.

IMMUNOMODULATORY PROPERTIES AND IMMUNOGENICITY OF MSCs IN VITRO AND IN VIVO

Tissue repair and disease improvement mediated by MSCs have been shown to be intimately related to MSC interaction with the host immune system in many disease models.[1,2] MSCs have clear immunomodulatory functions. It is increasingly recognized that the key to understanding MSC efficacy for tissue repair or inflammatory disease is to understand how MSCs modulate the inflammatory niche. MSCs have a distinct profile of bioactive mediators and adhesion molecules that work to inhibit scar formation, inhibit apoptosis, increase angiogenesis, and stimulate intrinsic progenitor cells to regenerate function. To accomplish this, MSCs interact with nearly all the cells of the immune system including lymphocyte B cells, T cells, natural killer (NK) cells, dendritic cells (DCs), macrophages/monocytes, and neutrophils,[3] suggesting far-reaching effects on early, innate, and humoral immune responses. It is unclear whether MSCs should be categorized as "immunosuppressive," implying a nonspecific downregulation of the immune system, or rather if they induce an "immune tolerance," implying a more specific suppression of aberrant immune responses. What does seem clear is that the immunomodulatory ability of MSCs is dependent on several factors including MSC activation, MSC tissue of origin, MSC dose, time of administration of MSCs, and MSC contact with cells of the immune system.

MSC Activation and Preconditioning

MSCs do not secrete immunomodulatory proteins in the absence of activation.[4,5] In vitro, activated T cells, individual or combinations of cytokines such as interferon-γ (IFN-γ) or tumor necrosis factor α (TNF-α), are used to activate MSCs.[5] In vivo, injected MSCs will become activated by the local inflammatory milieu, which is one reason why it is so critical to understand the inflammatory niche into which MSCs are injected. Acute injury characterized by interleukin (IL)-6, IL-1, or TNF-α would activate MSCs differently to chronic or immune-mediated lesions characterized by activated T cells or IFN-γ.

Recent evidence suggests that preconditioning of MSCs may enhance their survival and, as a result, enhance their regenerative and immunomodulatory properties.[6,7] In fact, research efforts within the field of regenerative therapy have been dedicated to understanding the in vitro manipulation of cells prior to transplantation, in an attempt to maximize their biological and functional properties.[8,9] Examples of these efforts include the use specific bioscaffolds that allow spatial and physical cell manipulation, increase cell survival, and promote integration with the host. Furthermore, culture strategies have been evaluated to improve MSC viability by exposing cells to hypoxic conditions,[10] specific growth factors,[11,12] or a variety of biological agents.[13]

Bone marrow (BM)-derived MSCs effectively migrate toward and enhance the healing processes that follow cardiac infarction and hind limb ischemia, both of which are characterized by a hypoxic gradient.[14–16] Although there is controversy regarding the effects of low oxygen tension on MSC survival, it appears that hypoxic conditions (1%–3% O_2) may be beneficial, as this oxygen tension is more similar to the physiologic niche of MSCs in the bone marrow (2%–7% O_2).[10] MSCs appear to maintain their viability and increase their proliferation rate when cultured in low oxygen tension environments.[10] These studies may provide support for the use of MSCs in the treatment of equine tendonitis. Tendon injuries are characterized by hypoxic degeneration, which leads to tenocyte apoptosis, particularly in chronic injury.[17,18] This hypoxic environment may be beneficial for MSC survival and may enhance their tissue-regenerating potential.

Pretreatment of MSCs with bioactive compounds in vitro, such as growth factors, may decrease cell death and promote cell replication. It is likely that a similar phenomenon takes place in vivo. Based on such studies, the use of platelet-rich plasma as a pretreatment medium and a cell delivery vehicle may be of value. Depending on the disease condition and pending the results of similar research conducted in horses, MSCs could be pretreated with bioactive compounds to allow them to survive longer and enhance their performance in vivo.

MSC Tissue of Origin

In humans and rodents, the ability of MSCs to alter the immune system varies with the MSC tissue of origin. MSCs can be harvested from numerous tissues and locations, and may have similar surface markers and growth characteristics; however, these MSCs display distinct differences.[19] Some studies, including the authors' own published studies,[20] suggest that BM-MSCs and adipose-derived MSCs (ASCs) are more closely related than to MSCs derived from placental tissues.[20,21] In humans, cord blood–derived MSCs express genes involved in the cell cycle and in neurogenesis, consistent with their reported neuronal differentiation capacity; BM-MSCs appear to be primed toward developmental processes of tissues and organs derived from the mesoderm and endoderm; and ASCs are highly enriched in immune-related genes.[21] These inherent differences appear to be further enhanced by inflammation. These transcriptome studies are compatible with in vitro tissue source comparison studies[22–24] showing that baseline and activated MSCs from BM, cord tissue, and ASC modulate the immune response and respond to inflammatory mediators distinctly.[5,25] Although research with MSCs from different tissue sources in horses is just beginning, equine MSCs appear to be remarkably similar to other species described to date. For example, equine MSCs derived from fat, BM, cord blood, and cord tissue all respond to activating stimuli such as TNF-α with the secretion of prostaglandin E_2 (PGE$_2$); however, secretion of other mediators, such as nitric oxide (NO), may be dependent on tissue of origin (Borjesson, unpublished data). It is critical to define mediators associated with immunomodulation for all animal species individually, as it is clear that there are strong interspecies differences in MSC responses to activation. For example, rodent MSCs and human MSCs differ slightly in their modulatory potential and mediators.[26]

MSC Dose

The inhibitory effects of MSCs are dose dependent. MSCs act on unstimulated T cells by preventing their activation. However, when T cells are already stimulated, MSCs reduce the expression levels of their activation markers. Some studies have shown that high doses of MSCs possess immunosuppressive activity whereas low-dose MSC therapy could be immunostimulatory[27,28] or fail to inhibit lymphocyte proliferation.[29,30] One study directly assessed MSC dose in a canine disc degeneration model and found that MSCs were least viable after injection at a low dose (10^5) and that there were more apoptotic cells at the high dose of MSCs (10^7), whereas the structural microenvironment and extracellular matrix of the disc were maintained with an intermediate dose of MSCs (10^6).[31] The ideal dose of MSCs for any given equine lesion is clearly an important area of study, and the dual ability of MSC to either sustain or suppress T-cell proliferation should be considered in the context of clinical applications.[28]

Time of Administration of MSC

There is very little information as to when MSCs should be administered, although some animal models support a time frame of 1 week post injury, after the acute inflammatory response recedes.[32,33] MSCs have shown dissimilar effects when applied at different stages of disease. As the inflammatory niche progresses from acute to chronic inflammation, the cells and mediators present could skew MSC activation in several ways. For example, in one study MSCs exhibited their typical suppressive phenotype when added early to cell cultures in the presence of CD4[+] T-cell polarizing stimuli. However, once T-cell activation had occurred, MSCs showed an opposite stimulating effect on Th17 cells, while leaving T-regulatory (Treg) IL-10–producing cells unchanged.[34] These results suggest that the therapeutic use of MSCs in vivo might exert opposing effects on disease activity, according to the time of therapeutic application and the level of effector T-cell activation, especially in autoimmune disease models.[34]

MSC Contact with Cells of the Immune System

MSCs act as pleiotropic immune regulators to suppress immune responses through the production of multiple soluble factors and/or direct cell-cell contact to affect all the actors of immune responses: T cells, NK cells, B cells, and DCs.[4,28] MSCs may act locally; however, they may also accumulate in secondary lymphoid organs and attenuate delayed-type hypersensitivity response by inducing apoptotic cell death of surrounding immune cells in the draining lymph node. In one study, MSCs accumulated in lymph nodes, near the paracortical area and the germinal center, and markedly attenuated a delayed-type hypersensitivity response via increased apoptosis of activated T cells.[35]

T lymphocytes

MSCs interact with T cells in several ways. MSCs secrete soluble mediators and directly interact with T cells to modulate their activity.[29,36,37] MSCs can induce apoptosis of activated T cells, induce cell-cycle arrest, decrease T-cell proliferation,[30,38] and alter T-cell phenotype. MSCs target T-cell subsets (CD4[+], CD8[+], CD2[+], and CD3[+] subpopulations) equally.[30] MSCs in direct contact with lymphocytes may inhibit lymphocyte apoptosis via the secretion of IL-6 or NO.[35–37] MSCs activated by IFN-γ upregulate adhesion molecules, including intracellular adhesion molecule 1 (CD54; ICAM-1) and vascular cell adhesion molecule 1 (CD106; VCAM-1).[37] In many models, direct contact between MSCs and T cells facilitates MSC immunosuppressive capacity. This direct association is presumed to facilitate the actions of locally produced, short-acting mediators such as NO.[37]

Decreased lymphocyte proliferation

For murine and human MSCs, the ability of MSCs to inhibit T-cell proliferation has been attributed to a variety of soluble mediators, adhesion molecules, and matrix metalloproteinases. Soluble mediators are also critical for the ability of equine MSCs to inhibit lymphocyte proliferation (Borjesson, unpublished data). Soluble factors reported to suppress T-cell proliferation include: PGE$_2$, hepatic growth factor, transforming growth factor β (TGF-β), IFN-γ, IL-10, leukemia inhibitory factor (LIF), human leukocyte antigen G (HLA-G), and indoleamine 2,3-dioxygenase (IDO).[4,28,30,38–42] MSC-derived matrix metalloproteinases can also cleave the IL-2 receptor (CD25) from the surface of activated T cells with a resultant reduction of IL-2 production.[35,43] This decreased production of IL-2 and IFN-γ, mediated by the NF-κB signaling pathway, also results in decreased lymphocyte proliferation.[35,43] MSC activation or priming by IFN-γ, TNF-α, and other proinflammatory cytokines increases their inhibitory effect (**Fig. 1**).[28]

Altered lymphocyte phenotype

MSCs are thought to induce lymphocytes to switch to a Treg phenotype (CD4[+]CD25[+]forkhead box P3 [FoxP3[+]] cells[28,39,44–47]). Tregs are a specialized subpopulation of T cells that suppress activation of the immune system and promote tolerance to self-antigens. In humans and mice, MSC-derived IDO, IL-10, PGE$_2$, and TGF-β have been implicated in the induction of Tregs.[39,45,47] Tregs are at least partially responsible for the anti-inflammatory Th1-dominant to Th2-dominant cytokine switch.[44] For human MSC-mediated allosuppression, some data support a sequential process of Treg induction involving direct MSC contact with CD4[+] cells followed by both PGE$_2$ and TGF-β expression.[45] Interest in Tregs is increasing as data from mouse models demonstrate that these cells may be responsible for MSC efficacy in the treatment of autoimmune diseases and may facilitate allograft (transplantation) tolerance.[39] Equine Tregs are being defined[48,49]; however, the study of Tregs in the context of equine MSCs and a lymphocyte-phenotype switch to Tregs has not yet been published.

Dendritic cells

In humans and rodents, MSCs also modulate DC maturation, differentiation, and function.[42,50,51] To date there are no reports of MSC interaction with equine DCs. The ability of DCs to initiate an immune response depends on their transition from an antigen-processing to an antigen-presenting cell. During this transition, major histocompatibility complex (MHC) class II and costimulatory molecules (CD80 and CD86) are upregulated on the cell surface, a process termed DC maturation. This

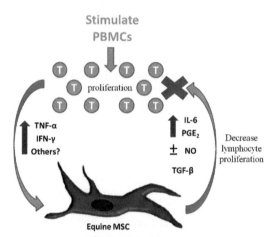

Fig. 1. Proposed model for immunomodulation by equine mesenchymal stem cells (MSCs). Stimulation of peripheral blood mononuclear cells (PBMCs), with a T-cell mitogen or nonself cells, causes T-cell proliferation and production of tumor necrosis factor α (TNF-α) and interferon-γ (IFN-γ). These cytokines activate the MSCs. Activated MSCs then produce immune-modulating cytokines including transforming growth factor β (TGF-β), interleukin-6 (IL-6), and prostaglandin E$_2$ (PGE$_2$), and variably produce nitric oxide (NO). These cytokines then act on the lymphocytes to decrease their proliferation. The mechanisms of this immunomodulation (eg, mediators responsible for reducing T-cell proliferation and the underlying mechanisms resulting in activation of MSCs and resultant alterations in T-cell proliferation) are still being elucidated. (*Courtesy of* Danielle D. Carrade, BS, Davis, CA, USA.)

transition is critical for mounting an immune response because immature DCs fail to prime T cells effectively, but induce tolerance rather than immune rejection. MSCs appear to keep DCs in an immature state,[51] and inhibit the maturation of myeloid-DCs and plasmocytoid-DCs.[42] MSCs also promote proliferation of mature DCs into a more immature "regulatory" phenotype.[51,52] DCs also interact with B cells and NK cells.[52] Similar to the themes described for T cells, MSC interaction with DCs depends on cell concentration, mechanism of activation, and the cohort of immune cells present. MSC modulation of DC function and maturation involves soluble factors, such as PGE_2, IL-6, or TGF-β, or cell-cell contact, or both.[42]

B lymphocytes

In humans and rodents, MSCs promote the survival and inhibit the proliferation and maturation of B cells by arresting them in the G_0/G_1 phase of the cell cycle.[53] MSCs also induce both stimulation and impairment of immunoglobulin production by B cells without affecting costimulatory molecule expression and cytokine production.[54,55] As with their interaction with all types of immune cells (T cells and DCs), MSC immuno-modulatory effects were dependent on the level of MSC activation (lipopolysaccharide or viral antigens) and whether MSCs were acting directly on (in contact with) unfractio-nated lymphocytes or enriched B cells.[55] The interaction of equine MSCs with B cells has not yet been reported.

Natural killer cells

NK cells are the major effectors of innate immunity, and their function is also inhibited by MSCs. MSCs alter NK cell phenotype, suppress cytokine-induced proliferation of NK cells, and prevent the induction of effector functions.[56,57] MSCs inhibit both NK cell–mediated cytolysis and IFN-γ secretion.[41] The inhibition of NK cell function is thought to be critical to the suppressive functions of MSCs, especially in therapeutic arenas such as graft-versus-host disease.[41]

MSC Secretion of Soluble Factors

As is clear from the preceding discussion, MSCs mediate their effects via direct cell-cell contact with cells of the immune system and via the secretion of soluble factors that also act on immune cell populations. There is a plethora of mediators that have been studied.[1,2] These mediators appear to act in concert (eg, with chemokines and adhesion molecules) or they may act sequentially. Many of the mediators have redundant roles (and their roles may be determined by the inflammatory lesion), but others may act as sole effectors of a particular anti-inflammatory response. In some cases, cell-cell contact may dictate the types of mediators secreted. For example, in the absence of cell-cell contact, MSC-induced expression of the tolerogenic genes IDO, LIF, and HLA-G does not occur.[40] However, when MSCs were able to directly contact T cells, the expression of IL-10 and TGF-β were modulated.[40] Activated equine MSCs produce abundant PGE_2 and IL-6 and variable amounts of NO and TGF-β, depending on tissue source and activation stimuli (Carrade and colleagues, in review). The significance of mediator secretion by equine MSCs has not been deter-mined (see **Fig. 1**).

Indoleamine 2,3-dioxygenase

Human MSCs express the tryptophan-catabolizing enzyme IDO, known to suppress T-cell responses.[4,5,26] IDO has been implicated in the induction of tolerogenic DCs, the switch to a Th2-dominant cytokine inflammatory response, and the induction of Tregs. In short, IDO is thought to be a central mediator in almost all aspects of MSC interaction with cells of the human immune system and induction of immune tolerance. Inhibition of IDO in allograft receipts resulted in an inability to achieve allo-graft tolerance.[39]

Human leukocyte antigens

MSCs from all species described to date, including horses,[58] express MHC I but do not express MHC II. The regulation of MHC I and MHC II (or HLA, the nomenclature of human MHC) on MSC can be altered by activation. Increased MHC can increase the immunogenicity of MSCs, for example by upregulation of HLA class I (MHC I) or HLA-DR (MHC II) expression.[5] Conversely, MSC activation by IFN-γ can enhance the immunosuppressive phenotype of MSCs by downregulating MHC II (HLA-DR) expression and increasing IDO production. Similarly, increased intracellular HLA-G and surface HLA-E expression can induce immune tolerance by increasing TGF-β and IL-10 release, and inducing IDO expression. MSCs have also been shown to secrete a soluble isoform of HLA class I molecule (HLA-G). This secretion is IL-10 dependent and requires cell-cell contact between MSCs and allostimulated T cells. HLA-G5 contributes to the suppression of allogeneic T-cell proliferation and then to the expansion of Tregs.[41] At present, very little is known about the family of MHC molecules in horses and how MHC regulation may contribute to MSC immunomodu-lation in horses.

CLINICAL IMPRESSIONS AND FUTURE IMPLICATIONS

Evidence suggests that MSCs play a role in cell survival and function in vivo. In labo-ratory animals with experimentally induced autoimmune encephalomyelitis, MSCs administered during hematopoietic stem cell transplantation MSC coadministration improves clinical outcomes by reducing the symptoms associated with grade 4 graft-versus-host response.[59] Similarly, there are many examples of a beneficial effect of MSCs in increasing the acceptability of coinfused hematopoietic stem cells and lessening the risk of graft-versus-host disease in people.[60–62] MSCs also enhance the longevity of cotransplanted MHC-incompatible skin grafts in baboons.[63,64] These studies indicate the need to expand the scientific knowledge and the use of MSCs in horses beyond regenerative applications. MSCs could be applied in chronic wound management whereby a dysregulation of the healing process creates an aberrant inflammatory and resultant hyperplastic response such as that seen with exuberant granulation tissue in horses. The authors have infused autologous MSCs via intrave-nous regional limb perfusion in 3 horses with "proud flesh," and have observed encouraging healing responses. In these horses, intravenous infusions of 20×10^6 MSCs suspended in physiologic solution were performed for 3 consecutive days. Although traditional therapeutic strategies had previously failed, these wounds continued to be treated with standard medical approaches such as bandaging and surgical debridement.

The use of banked MSCs obtained from donor horses offers the advantage of an expeditious treatment as well as the use of an established and homogenous cell pop-ulation with proven regenerative and differentiation capacity. Allogeneic BM-MSCs (obtained from donor animals) may have inhibitory and antiproliferative effects on T-cell and B-cell function similar to that seen in a murine model of systemic lupus erythematosus with spontaneous and lethal autoimmune responses.[65] Other diseases in which conventional immunosuppressive therapies fail may provide a rationale for the use of MSC-based therapeutic approaches.[66–68] MSC infusions may also play an important role in regulating inflammatory diseases of the central nervous system, although their interactions with the blood-brain barrier have not been fully elucidated.[67,69,70]

Studies aimed at assessing the efficacy and safety of allogeneic treatments in horses are lacking, although pilot studies have shown that inflammatory cell infiltration was no different in surgically induced equine superficial digital flexor tendon lesions, regardless of whether MSCs were allogeneic or autologous.[71] Furthermore, injection of allogeneic placentally derived MSCs into equine joints resulted in self-limiting inflammatory responses, with no difference in the type or severity of the inflammatory response elicited by autologous versus allogeneic MSCs.[58]

The authors' clinical impressions resulting from treating horses with intravenous or intralesional injections of allogeneic BM-MSCs have been generally positive. Several horses within the authors' respective institutions have been treated with banked BM-derived MSCs for a variety of hard and soft tissue disorders, such as osteochondrosis, osteoarthritis, and tendonitis. Local reactions have been self-limiting and easily treated with the administration of nonsteroidal anti-inflammatory medications. It is interesting that some of the best responses to the cell therapy were seen in those horses in which a reaction was observed following the intralesional injection. Large-scale prospective studies are needed to optimize cell-based therapy in horses. These studies would ideally provide answers to key questions such as the route of administration, the appropriate cell dose, and the necessary control required to determine the value of the selected cell therapy.

REFERENCES

1. Griffin MD, Ritter T, Mahon BP. Immunological aspects of allogeneic mesenchymal stem cell therapies. Hum Gene Ther 2010;21(12):1641–55.
2. Singer NG, Caplan AI. Mesenchymal stem cells: mechanisms of inflammation. Annu Rev Pathol 2011;6:457–78.
3. Brandau S, Jakob M, Hemeda H, et al. Tissue-resident mesenchymal stem cells attract peripheral blood neutrophils and enhance their inflammatory activity in response to microbial challenge. J Leukoc Biol 2010;88(5):1005–15.
4. DelaRosa O, Lombardo E, Beraza A, et al. Requirement of IFN-gamma-mediated indoleamine 2,3-dioxygenase expression in the modulation of lymphocyte proliferation by human adipose-derived stem cells. Tissue Eng Part A 2009;15(10): 2795–806.
5. Deuse T, Stubbendorff M, Tang-Quan K, et al. Immunogenicity and immunomodulatory properties of umbilical cord lining mesenchymal stem cells. Cell Transplant 2010.
6. Cheng AS, Yau TM. Paracrine effects of cell transplantation: strategies to augment the efficacy of cell therapies. Semin Thorac Cardiovasc Surg 2008; 20(2):94–101.
7. Shihab FS. Preconditioning: from experimental findings to novel therapies in acute kidney injury. Minerva Urol Nefrol 2009;61(3):143–57.
8. Herrmann JL, Wang Y, Abarbanell AM, et al. Preconditioning mesenchymal stem cells with transforming growth factor-alpha improves mesenchymal stem cell-mediated cardioprotection. Shock 2010;33(1):24–30.
9. Gyongyosi M, Posa A, Pavo N, et al. Differential effect of ischaemic preconditioning on mobilisation and recruitment of haematopoietic and mesenchymal stem cells in porcine myocardial ischaemia-reperfusion. Thromb Haemost 2010;104(2):376–84.
10. Rosova I, Dao M, Capoccia B, et al. Hypoxic preconditioning results in increased motility and improved therapeutic potential of human mesenchymal stem cells. Stem Cells 2008;26(8):2173–82.

11. Khan M, Akhtar S, Mohsin S, et al. Growth factor preconditioning increases the function of diabetes-impaired mesenchymal stem cells. Stem Cells Dev 2011; 20(1):67–75.

12. Mias C, Trouche E, Seguelas MH, et al. Ex vivo pretreatment with melatonin improves survival, proangiogenic/mitogenic activity, and efficiency of mesenchymal stem cells injected into ischemic kidney. Stem Cells 2008;26(7):1749–57.

13. Wang ZJ, Zhang FM, Wang LS, et al. Lipopolysaccharides can protect mesenchymal stem cells (MSCs) from oxidative stress-induced apoptosis and enhance proliferation of MSCs via Toll-like receptor (TLR)-4 and PI3K/Akt. Cell Biol Int 2009;33(6):665–74.

14. Pittenger MF, Martin BJ. Mesenchymal stem cells and their potential as cardiac therapeutics. Circ Res 2004;95(1):9–20.

15. Shake JG, Gruber PJ, Baumgartner WA, et al. Mesenchymal stem cell implantation in a swine myocardial infarct model: engraftment and functional effects. Ann Thorac Surg 2002;73(6):1919–25 [discussion: 1926].

16. Nakagami H, Maeda K, Morishita R, et al. Novel autologous cell therapy in ischemic limb disease through growth factor secretion by cultured adipose tissue-derived stromal cells. Arterioscler Thromb Vasc Biol 2005;25(12):2542–7.

17. Benson RT, McDonnell SM, Knowles, et al. Tendinopathy and tears of the rotator cuff are associated with hypoxia and apoptosis. J Bone Joint Surg Br 2010;92(3): 448–53.

18. Kannus P, Jozsa L. Histopathological changes preceding spontaneous rupture of a tendon. A controlled study of 891 patients. J Bone Joint Surg Am 1991;73(10): 1507–25.

19. Chang HY, Chi JT, Dudoit S, et al. Diversity, topographic differentiation, and positional memory in human fibroblasts. Proc Natl Acad Sci U S A 2002;99(20): 12877–82.

20. Toupadakis CA, Wong A, Genetos DC, et al. Comparison of the osteogenic potential of equine mesenchymal stem cells from bone marrow, adipose tissue, umbilical cord blood, and umbilical cord tissue. Am J Vet Res 2010;71(10): 1237–45.

21. Jansen BJ, Gilissen C, Roelofs H, et al. Functional differences between mesenchymal stem cell populations are reflected by their transcriptome. Stem Cells Dev 2010;19(4):481–90.

22. Kern S, Eichler H, Stoeve J, et al. Comparative analysis of mesenchymal stem cells from bone marrow, umbilical cord blood, or adipose tissue. Stem Cells 2006;24(5):1294–301.

23. Keyser KA, Beagles KE, Kiem HP. Comparison of mesenchymal stem cells from different tissues to suppress T-cell activation. Cell Transplant 2007;16(5):555–62.

24. Yoo KH, Jang IK, Lee MW, et al. Comparison of immunomodulatory properties of mesenchymal stem cells derived from adult human tissues. Cell Immunol 2009; 259(2):150–6.

25. Prasanna SJ, Gopalakrishnan D, Shankar SR, et al. Pro-inflammatory cytokines, IFNgamma and TNFalpha, influence immune properties of human bone marrow and Wharton jelly mesenchymal stem cells differentially. PLoS One 2010;5(2): e9016.

26. Ren G, Su J, Zhang L, et al. Species variation in the mechanisms of mesenchymal stem cell-mediated immunosuppression. Stem Cells 2009;27(8):1954–62.

27. Sun B, Zhang X, Wang G. Regulation of suppressing and activating effects of mesenchymal stem cells on the encephalitogenic potential of MBP68-86-specific lymphocytes. J Neuroimmunol 2010;226(1–2):116–25.

28. Najar M, Rouas R, Raicevic G, et al. Mesenchymal stromal cells promote or suppress the proliferation of T lymphocytes from cord blood and peripheral blood: the importance of low cell ratio and role of interleukin-6. Cytotherapy 2009;11(5): 570–83.

29. Najar M, Raicevic G, Id Boufker H, et al. Modulated expression of adhesion molecules and galectin-1: role during mesenchymal stromal cell immunoregulatory functions. Exp Hematol 2010;38(10):922–32.

30. Najar M, Raicevic G, Boufker HI, et al. Mesenchymal stromal cells use PGE2 to modulate activation and proliferation of lymphocyte subsets: combined comparison of adipose tissue, Wharton's Jelly and bone marrow sources. Cell Immunol 2010;264(2):171–9.

31. Serigano K, Sakai D, Hiyama A, et al. Effect of cell number on mesenchymal stem cell transplantation in a canine disc degeneration model. J Orthop Res 2010; 28(10):1267–75.

32. Han SS, Kweon OK. Comparison of canine umbilical cord blood-derived mesenchymal stem cell transplantation times: Involvement of astrogliosis, inflammation, intracellular actin cytoskeleton pathways, and neurotrophin. Cell Transplant 2011. [Epub ahead of print]. DOI: 10.3727/096368911X566163.

33. Hu X, Wang J, Chen J. Optimal temporal delivery of bone marrow mesenchymal stem cells in rats with myocardial infarction. Eur J Cardiothorac Surg 2007;31(3): 438–43.

34. Carrion F, Nova E, Luz P, et al. Opposing effect of mesenchymal stem cells on Th1 and Th17 cell polarization according to the state of CD4(+) T cell activation. Immunol Lett 2011;135(1–2):10–6.

35. Lim JH, Kim JS, Yoon IH, et al. Immunomodulation of delayed-type hypersensitivity responses by mesenchymal stem cells is associated with bystander T cell apoptosis in the draining lymph node. J Immunol 2010;185(7):4022–9.

36. Xu G, Zhang Y, Zhang L, et al. The role of IL-6 in inhibition of lymphocyte apoptosis by mesenchymal stem cells. Biochem Biophys Res Commun 2007; 361(3):745–50.

37. Ren G, Zhao X, Zhang L. Inflammatory cytokine-induced intercellular adhesion molecule-1 and vascular cell adhesion molecule-1 in mesenchymal stem cells are critical for immunosuppression. J Immunol 2010;184(5):2321–8.

38. Cui L, Yin S, Liu W, et al. Expanded adipose-derived stem cells suppress mixed lymphocyte reaction by secretion of prostaglandin E2. Tissue Eng 2007;13(6): 1185–95.

39. Ge W, Jiang J, Arp J, et al. Regulatory T-cell generation and kidney allograft tolerance induced by mesenchymal stem cells associated with indoleamine 2,3-dioxygenase expression. Transplantation 2010;90(12):1312–20.

40. Nasef A, Chapel A, Mazurier C, et al. Identification of IL-10 and TGF-beta transcripts involved in the inhibition of T-lymphocyte proliferation during cell contact with human mesenchymal stem cells. Gene Expr 2007;13(4–5):217–26.

41. Selmani Z, Naji A, Zidi I, et al. Human leukocyte antigen-G5 secretion by human mesenchymal stem cells is required to suppress T lymphocyte and natural killer function and to induce CD4+CD25highFOXP3+ regulatory T cells. Stem Cells 2008;26(1):212–22.

42. Yanez R, Oviedo A, Aldea M, et al. Prostaglandin E2 plays a key role in the immunosuppressive properties of adipose and bone marrow tissue-derived mesenchymal stromal cells. Exp Cell Res 2010;316(19):3109–23.

43. Shi D, Liao L, Zhang B, et al. Human adipose tissue-derived mesenchymal stem cells facilitate the immunosuppressive effect of cyclosporin A on T lymphocytes

through Jagged-1-mediated inhibition of NF-kappaB signaling. Exp Hematol 2011;39(2):214.e1–24.e1.

44. Di Ianni M, Del Papa B, De Ioanni M, et al. Mesenchymal cells recruit and regulate T regulatory cells. Exp Hematol 2008;36(3):309–18.

45. English K, Ryan JM, Tobin L, et al. Cell contact, prostaglandin E(2) and transforming growth factor beta 1 play non-redundant roles in human mesenchymal stem cell induction of CD4+CD25(High) forkhead box P3+ regulatory T cells. Clin Exp Immunol 2009;156(1):149–60.

46. Li H, Guo ZK, Li XS, et al. Functional and phenotypic alteration of intrasplenic lymphocytes affected by mesenchymal stem cells in a murine allosplenocyte transfusion model. Cell Transplant 2007;16(1):85–95.

47. Madec AM, Mallone R, Afonso G, et al. Mesenchymal stem cells protect NOD mice from diabetes by inducing regulatory T cells. Diabetologia 2009;52(7): 1391–9.

48. Banham AH, Lyne L, Scase TJ, et al. Monoclonal antibodies raised to the human FOXP3 protein can be used effectively for detecting Foxp3(+) T cells in other mammalian species. Vet Immunol Immunopathol 2009;127(3–4):376–81.

49. Robbin MG, Wagner B, Noronha LE, et al. Subpopulations of equine blood lymphocytes expressing regulatory T cell markers. Vet Immunol Immunopathol 2011;140(1–2):90–101.

50. Nauta AJ, Kruisselbrink AB, Lurvink E, et al. Mesenchymal stem cells inhibit generation and function of both CD34+-derived and monocyte-derived dendritic cells. J Immunol 2006;177(4):2080–7.

51. Li YP, Paczesny S, Lauret E, et al. Human mesenchymal stem cells license adult CD34+ hemopoietic progenitor cells to differentiate into regulatory dendritic cells through activation of the Notch pathway. J Immunol 2008;180(3):1598–608.

52. Zhang B, Liu R, Shi D, et al. Mesenchymal stem cells induce mature dendritic cells into a novel Jagged-2-dependent regulatory dendritic cell population. Blood 2009;113(1):46–57.

53. Tabera S, Perez-Simon JA, Diez-Campelo M, et al. The effect of mesenchymal stem cells on the viability, proliferation and differentiation of B-lymphocytes. Haematologica 2008;93(9):1301–9.

54. Corcione A, Benvenuto F, Ferretti E, et al. Human mesenchymal stem cells modulate B-cell functions. Blood 2006;107(1):367–72.

55. Rasmusson I, Le Blanc K, Sundberg B, et al. Mesenchymal stem cells stimulate antibody secretion in human B cells. Scand J Immunol 2007;65(4):336–43.

56. Prigione I, Benvenuto F, Bocca P, et al. Reciprocal interactions between human mesenchymal stem cells and gammadelta T cells or invariant natural killer T cells. Stem Cells 2009;27(3):693–702.

57. Spaggiari GM, Capobianco A, Abdelrazik H, et al. Mesenchymal stem cells inhibit natural killer-cell proliferation, cytotoxicity, and cytokine production: role of indoleamine 2,3-dioxygenase and prostaglandin E2. Blood 2008;111(3):1327–33.

58. Carrade DD, Owens SD, Galuppo LD, et al. Clinicopathologic findings following intra-articular injection of autologous and allogeneic placentally derived equine mesenchymal stem cells in horses. Cytotherapy 2011;13(4):419–30.

59. Zappia E, Casazza S, Pedemonte E, et al. Mesenchymal stem cells ameliorate experimental autoimmune encephalomyelitis inducing T-cell anergy. Blood 2005;106(5):1755–61.

60. Wang RP, Chen H, Guo YQ, et al. Research progress on immunologic mechanisms of mesenchymal stem cells for treatment of graft-versus-host disease. Zhongguo Shi Yan Xue Ye Xue Za Zhi 2011;19(2):550–3 [in Chinese].

61. Vemuri MC, Chase LG, Rao MS. Mesenchymal stem cell assays and applications. Methods Mol Biol 2011;698:3–8.
62. Ringden O, Le Blanc K. Mesenchymal stem cells for treatment of acute and chronic graft-versus-host disease, tissue toxicity and hemorrhages. Best Pract Res Clin Haematol 2011;24(1):65–72.
63. Bartholomew A, Sturgeon C, Siatskas M, et al. Mesenchymal stem cells suppress lymphocyte proliferation in vitro and prolong skin graft survival in vivo. Exp Hematol 2002;30(1):42–8.
64. Krampera M, Franchini M, Pizzolo G, et al. Mesenchymal stem cells: from biology to clinical use. Blood Transfus 2007;5(3):120–9.
65. Deng W, Han Q, Liao L, et al. Effects of allogeneic bone marrow-derived mesenchymal stem cells on T and B lymphocytes from BXSB mice. DNA Cell Biol 2005; 24(7):458–63.
66. Jorgensen C, Djouad F, Apparailly F, et al. Engineering mesenchymal stem cells for immunotherapy. Gene Ther 2003;10(10):928–31.
67. Joyce N, Annett G, Wirthlin L, et al. Mesenchymal stem cells for the treatment of neurodegenerative disease. Regen Med 2010;5(6):933–46.
68. Ko IK, Kim BG, Awadallah A, et al. Targeting improves MSC treatment of inflammatory bowel disease. Mol Ther 2010;18(7):1365–72.
69. Ichim TE, Solano F, Glenn E, et al. Stem cell therapy for autism. J Transl Med 2007;5:30.
70. Theus MH, Wei L, Cui L, et al. In vitro hypoxic preconditioning of embryonic stem cells as a strategy of promoting cell survival and functional benefits after transplantation into the ischemic rat brain. Exp Neurol 2008;210(2):656–70.
71. Smith RK. Mesenchymal stem cell therapy for equine tendinopathy. Disabil Rehabil 2008;30(20–22):1752–8.

Commercial Cell-based Therapies for Musculoskeletal Injuries in Horses

Santiago D. Gutierrez-Nibeyro, DVM, MS

KEYWORDS

- Bone marrow–derived mesenchymal stem cells
- Bone marrow aspirate concentrate
- Adipose tissue–derived stromal vascular fraction cells
- Embryonic-like stem cells

Equine veterinary practitioners currently have several commercial cell-based therapeutic options available to treat musculoskeletal injuries in horses. Although there is limited research in this area, the current literature supports the use of cell-based therapies to treat equine musculoskeletal injuries. As the field of cell-based regenerative medicine develops, researchers continue to search for more effective cell-based therapies to provide practitioners with optimal treatment tools for musculoskeletal injuries encountered by horses. Cell-based therapies require specialized facilities and technical competencies that might not be available or economically justifiable in many private practices. This review provides a brief summary of the current commercially available cell-based therapeutic products for equine applications, their similarities and differences, and current objective data relating to their clinical efficacy.

COMMERCIAL CELL-BASED THERAPIES FOR MUSCULOSKELETAL INJURIES IN HORSES

The use of cell-based therapies for musculoskeletal injuries in horses is becoming widely accepted among equine practitioners in North America. The goal of these "biological" therapies is to enhance regeneration of injured or diseased tissues that regenerate poorly, such as tendon, ligaments, menisci, and cartilage.[1] Although the capacity of these novel therapies to restore the normal structure and mechanical properties of the original tissue is debatable at this stage, there is growing scientific evidence that supports the use of cell-based therapies to improve healing of

---

The author has nothing to disclose.
Department of Clinical Veterinary Medicine, College of Veterinary Medicine, University of Illinois, 1008 West Hazelwood Drive, Champaign-Urbana, IL 61802, USA
E-mail address: sgn@illinois.edu

musculoskeletal injuries in horses. In fact, it appears that intralesional administration of stem cells may enhance intrinsic healing,[2,3] minimize initial inflammation and scarring,[4,5] and decrease the re-injury rate of superficial digital flexor tendinopathy in horses.[6,7] Quite apart from issues related to clinical efficacy, biological therapies have distinct advantages in performance horses in that they are not subject to "drug detection" and withholding restrictions that pertain to the administration of pharmaceutical agents.

It is well established that equine mesenchymal stem cells (MSCs) are capable of differentiating into fibroblasts, osteoblasts, or chondroblasts in vitro.[5,8–16] However, the current difficulty in using MSCs for clinical applications relates to our inability to reliably direct appropriate MSC differentiation in injured musculoskeletal tissues.[10,15] The definitive number of cells necessary to achieve a beneficial clinical effect is still unknown. Most in vivo work focused on the effect of "regenerative" cells in tendon injuries has showed promising results after intralesional injection of cell suspension containing 5×10^6 to 10×10^6 MSCs.[2,4,6,7] However, a recent study conducted in horses with collagenase-induced tendon injuries demonstrated that nonexpanded bone marrow aspirate and expanded bone marrow–derived MSCs were equally effective in improving tendon healing and extracellular matrix organization.[5] These results demonstrate that research is still necessary to identify the mechanisms of action of cell-based therapies and to determine the optimal number of MSCs needed to effectively treat specific musculoskeletal injuries.

At present most practitioners use autogenous cell-based products, but there is a large body of scientific evidence suggesting that allogenic embryonic-like stem cells (ESCs) and bone marrow–derived MSCs (BMDMSCs) can also be used without eliciting a detectable cell-mediated immune response in horses.[16,17] To date, a limited number of horses with soft tissue injuries have been treated with allogenic bone marrow–derived MSCs without detrimental clinical effects (J. Peroni, personal communication, 2010). This evidence suggests that allogenic cell-based products may be used in the near future for intralesional therapy immediately after diagnosis of acute injuries to overcome the practical limitations of autologous products. Additional research is necessary to determine the viability and effects of allogenic cell-based products in musculoskeletal injuries of horses before the clinical use of these therapies. This approach also has the potential to increase the risk of disease transfer to the patient.

CURRENT CELL-BASED THERAPIES FOR MUSCULOSKELETAL INJURIES IN HORSES

At present, practitioners have access to several commercial cell-based therapeutic options to treat musculoskeletal injuries in horses, including BMDMSCs, bone marrow aspirate concentrate (BMAC), adipose tissue–derived stromal vascular fraction cells (ADSVFCs), umbilical cord blood MSCs, and ESCs. Most of these therapies were initially available through university-based research laboratories. However, many of these therapies are now available through commercial laboratories in North America. At present, cultured BMDMSCs and ADSVFCs are the most commonly used cell-based products to enhance regeneration of diseased or injured musculoskeletal tissues in horses. Initial in vitro studies have demonstrated that equine BMDMSCs have a superior differentiation potential to adipose tissue-derived MSCs, which suggests that BMDMSCs are a superior source of cells for regeneration of musculoskeletal tissue in horses.[8,9,11,18] However, this difference has not yet been demonstrated in vivo studies, and the ease of adipose tissue collection represents a considerable advantage for most practitioners.

Bone Marrow–Derived Mesenchymal Stem Cells

The number of MSCs yielded from bone marrow aspirates is considered to be too low to elicit a primary regenerative effect. MSC numbers can be increased by a 2- to 3-week in vitro expansion prior to administration.[19] In the United States, there are several university research laboratories and two commercial laboratories that provide MSC isolation and expansion services from autologous bone marrow aspirates for veterinary use (**Table 1**).

One of these commercial laboratories is Advanced Regenerative Therapies (ART, Fort Collins, CO, USA), which originated from the Colorado State University Equine Orthopaedic Research Center. The company provides culture expansion of MSCs for treatment of intra-articular, tendon, and ligament injuries. Harvesting, shipping, and injection instructions can be found at www.art4dvm.com. In brief, a bone marrow aspirate is collected from the ilium or sternum and shipped to ART using a next-day courier. At ART, the MSCs are isolated from the sample and expanded to generate at least 5×10^6 to 15×10^6 cells (this is the company's recommended dose for clinical applications). This process typically requires 2 to 3 weeks. After in vitro expansion, the MSCs are cryopreserved and shipped on dry ice back to the practitioner for treatment.

The use of BMDMSCs is an attractive option for equine joint disease; however, in a recent study using the osteochondral fragment equine model of osteoarthritis, neither intra-articular injection of BMDMSCs (Equine Orthopaedic Research Center, Colorado State University, Fort Collins, CO, USA) or ADSVFCs (Vet-Stem, Poway, CA, USA) had a significant clinical effect compared with controls.[18] The results from the experimental model are in contrast to recent findings that demonstrated good outcomes in clinical cases treated with BMDMSCs. Of 40 horses with joint disease (the majority had subchondral bone cysts or meniscal injuries in one or both stifles), 29 (72%) returned to full work and 14 (35%) performed at a previous level following intra-articular BMDMSCs and rehabilitation.[20,21] Further work is necessary to establish whether, in fact, intra-articular BMDMSCs are effective in treating osteoarthritis in horses, but the results to date suggest that this therapy is useful for the treatment of arthritis involving the soft tissue structures of the stifle joint.

Table 1
Commercial sources of "regenerative cells" available for equine practitioners in North America

Company	Web Site	Product Sent	Product Returned	Turnaround
ART	www.art4dvm.com	Bone marrow aspirate	Bone marrow–derived MSCs	2–3 wk
VetCell Bioscience Ltd	www.vetcellamericas.com	Bone marrow aspirate	Bone marrow–derived MSCs	2–3 wk
Vet-Stem	www.vet-stem.com	Adipose tissue	Adipose tissue–derived stromal vascular fraction cells	48 h
EquStem	www.equstem.com	Umbilical cord blood	Umbilical cord blood–derived MSCs	Not available
EquStem	www.equstem.com	Bone marrow aspirate	Bone marrow-derived MSCs	2–3 wk
Celavet	www.celavet.com	Not applicable	Fetal-derived embryonic-like stem cells	Not available

VetCell (VetCell Bioscience Ltd, Oxfordshire, UK), a company that originated in partnership with the Royal Veterinary College to provide stem cell service to the veterinary market in Europe and Australia, has recently started to provide this service in the United States. The company (VetCell Bioscience Inc, Dawsonville, GA, USA) provides in vitro expansion of MSCs for treatment of tendon and ligament injuries through the Coriell Institute for Medical Research, using VetCell's patented technique. VetCell recommends treating tendon and ligament injuries with a minimum of 10×10^6 cells, which can be obtained within 2 to 3 weeks of in vitro expansion. After expansion, the cells are resuspended in autogenous bone marrow supernatant (to a final concentration of 5×10^6 cells/mL), preloaded into 1-mL syringes, and returned to the practitioner. In addition, the company also provides storage service for potential future treatments. Harvesting, shipping, and injection instructions can be found at www.vetcellamericas.com. Bone marrow aspiration kits and insulated transport containers can be obtained from MILA International (www.milainternational.com). In Canada, the VetCell stem cell service is available through the Atlantic Veterinary College at the University of Prince Edward Island.

According to the company, to date more than 1500 horses with soft tissue injuries have been treated worldwide with intralesional BMDMSCs generated by the VetCell technique. Analysis of the clinical outcome of 113 racehorses affected by superficial digital flexor tendinopathy revealed a lower re-injury rate following intralesional cell therapy when compared with horses with similar lesions that received the standard of care (27% and 57%, respectively).[22] These results are supported by a recent experimental study that showed improvement of mechanical, morphologic, and compositional parameters of naturally occurring superficial digital flexor tendinopathy treated with BMDMSCs.[22]

Bone Marrow Aspirate Concentrate

The use of autologous cultured MSCs to treat musculoskeletal injuries in horses can be costly and is not immediately available at the time of diagnosis. Therefore, the use of MSCs without an expansion step is an alternative therapeutic option in horses. Typically the bone marrow aspirate is centrifuged to concentrate platelets and mononucleated cells (containing MSCs) using a similar technique to that used to produce platelet-rich plasma.[3,23] Thus, the number of MSCs contained in bone marrow aspirates can be rapidly increased using a point-of-care device without an in vitro culture step. From a clinician's perspective, BMAC is a convenient cell-based therapy because it is relatively inexpensive, the processing technique is straightforward and rapid, minimal equipment is needed, and it allows point-of-care treatment. In addition, BMAC contains all 3 components for optimal tissue regeneration: scaffold, growth factors, and stem cells.[24] The biggest disadvantage of BMAC is the lower number of MSCs delivered per injection volume when compared with culture-expanded MSCs.[3]

There are several devices on the market for procuring BMAC for human use. However, only one system (SmartPReP2 BMAC System, Harvest Technologies, Plymouth, MA, USA) has been evaluated to concentrate platelets and bone marrow aspirate from dogs and horses.[3,23] The system includes process disposables, instructions, and other accessories to isolate and concentrate the MSC fraction in a reduced volume for intralesional injection (www.harvesttech.com). Cytologic analyses of equine BMAC have confirmed that the system can be used to increase both platelets and mononucleated cells in the bone marrow aspirate (8.7- and 7.4-fold, respectively) over baseline aspirates, with an estimated $13.4\% \pm 4\%$ of the mononucleated cells contained in the BMAC being MSCs.[3]

BMAC has been used to induce bone formation in humans with osseous defects, nonunions, or osteonecrosis.[25–28] In horses BMAC has been used to improve cartilage, bone, and tendon repair, with good results. Microfracture combined with BMAC resulted in superior cartilage repair in experimentally induced full-thickness cartilage defects, compared with that following microfracture alone.[3] Further, in a collagenase-induced model of superficial digital flexor tendonitis, BMAC-treated and BMDMSC-treated tendons had greater expression of cartilage oligomeric matrix protein, a higher collagen type I/III ratio, and a more longitudinally oriented fiber pattern than fibrin glue and saline-treated tendons.[5] Of interest, in the same study BMAC and BMDMSCs had similar effects on treated tendons, suggesting that both approaches may be effective for regeneration of tendon tissue in horses.

A recent clinical study reported that 21 of 32 (66%) horses with a deep digital flexor tendinopathy treated with intralesional BMAC or culture-expanded MSCs returned to full athletic use 12 months after treatment, with both treatments being equally effective.[29] This outcome was superior to the results from horses with similar injuries managed conservatively (28%).[30] Based on this evidence and the advantages of the use of BMAC in clinical practice, BMAC appears to be an excellent cell-based therapy for practitioners managing deep digital flexor tendinopathy. BMAC is also being used for intra-articular therapy, but no clinical data have been reported on its use as yet.

Adipose Tissue–Derived Stromal Vascular Fraction Cells

Vet-Stem (Regenerative Veterinary Medicine, Poway, CA, USA) is the only stem cell service that supplies ADSVFCs to the veterinary market in the United States. This laboratory uses a relatively simple technique to isolate a heterogeneous population of stromal vascular fraction cells (MSCs, endothelial progenitor cells, hematopoietic stem cells, fibroblasts, and others) from adipose tissue. This cell suspension can be used to treat intra-articular or tendon/ligament injuries immediately after diagnosis, or can be expanded in culture to yield adipose tissue–derived MSCs. Adipose tissue–derived stromal vascular fraction cells (Vet-Stem regenerative cells, VSRC) have been a popular source of "regenerative cells" for equine musculoskeletal injuries in North America, because a high number of nucleated cells with potential anti-inflammatory and regenerative effects are obtained from each sample within 24 to 48 hours of tissue collection.[4] However, it has been found that only 2% to 4% of the nucleated cells recovered from adipose tissue are "stem cells," which is far less than the number of MSCs obtained with bone marrow–derived, culture-expanded samples.[15] Current expert opinion holds that the current technique to isolate MSCs from adipose tissue results in a subtherapeutic number of MSCs for musculoskeletal therapy,[31] but the clinical significance of these data is unknown because there are no data that document the number of MSCs necessary to treat musculoskeletal injuries in horses.

Adipose tissue typically is harvested from the pericoccygeal region, although the sternal or inguinal regions can be used as donor sites if scarring on the tail head is cosmetically unacceptable. The sample is shipped to the company using a next-day courier. At the laboratory, the adipose tissue is digested and centrifuged to isolate the regenerative cells. The resulting stromal vascular cell fraction is resuspended in buffered physiologic solution and shipped to the veterinarian in 3 separate syringes (0.6 mL/syringe) containing between 10×10^6 and 17×10^6 cells in each syringe.[4,18] Harvesting, shipping, and injection instructions are provided on the Web site (www.vet-stem.com). In addition, the company provides culture expansion and storage of adipose tissue–derived cells for additional treatments of an existing injury, or for a possible future need. This protocol is supported by a recent publication that demonstrated that the total number of adipose tissue–derived MSCs can be rapidly expanded in culture.[15]

Adipose tissue–derived stromal vascular fraction cells have been used to improve tendon and ligament repair, with apparently good results. In a recent controlled in vivo study that compared intralesional ADSVFCs and saline solution in a collagenase-induced model of superficial digital flexor tendonitis, ADSVFC-treated tendons had significantly better histologic organization and reduced inflammatory cell infiltrate than controls at 6 weeks.[4] It should be noted that the study was funded by the same laboratory that provides stem cell service for veterinary use in the United States. This study is the only peer-reviewed publication that has investigated the effect of ADSVFCs in soft tissue injuries in horses.

A press release in December 2010 from Vet-Stem stated that more than 4000 horses have been treated with commercially processed ADSVFCs since 2004, without systemic adverse effects and less than 0.5% local tissue reactions after administration. Results of recent clinical studies evaluating the efficacy of ADSVFCs isolated by the Vet-Stem method are encouraging, and can be found at www.vet-stem.com. A summary of these results are presented here. Of 66 horses with tendon injuries treated with ADSVFCs, 62 (94%) returned to full work and 51 (77%) performed at their previous level. Also, of 52 horses with suspensory desmopathy treated with ADSVFCs, 94% returned to full work and the majority (77%) performed at their previous level.[32] In addition, the company claims that ADSVFCs are effective for the treatment of joint injuries, as 50 of 60 horses (83%) with joint injuries returned to full work and 34 (57%) performed at a previous level. It should be noted that all of the studies were performed by the company.

Information regarding the efficacy and safety of culture-expanded, adipose tissue–derived MSCs to treat musculoskeletal injuries in horses is limited at this point. However, a recent prospective study of racehorses that had superficial digital flexor tendinopathy (n = 18) or suspensory desmopathy (n = 40) treated with expanded adipose-derived MSCs reported that 32 of 53 horses (60%) returned to full athletic function, but 14 horses (26%) were re-injured at a 18- to 24-month follow-up.[33] Although this re-injury rate may seem high, 7 of 14 horses (50%) with re-injuries had previously injured the same tendon before stem cell treatment. Thus, only 7 horses with an injury initially treated with stem cells suffered a recurrent injury.[33]

Recently Stemlogix (Stemlogix LLC, Weston, FL, USA) has entered the veterinary market, providing veterinarians with the training, equipment, and supplies necessary to deliver ADSVFCs to patients as a point-of-care therapy. This company has developed techniques and kits necessary to isolate nucleated cell fractions from a patient's adipose tissue directly on-site at their own clinic. This technique allows clinicians to obtain a relatively high pool of cells ready for delivery to the patient within 60 to 90 minutes of harvest.

According to data provided by the company, more than 90% of the cells are viable at point of care while cell viability decreases by 40% for processed cells kept outside the body for 24 hours. The initial investment for equipment and supplies necessary to process the samples and isolate cells is between $5000 and $10,000 depending on each individual clinic's equipment needs. The kits to process samples from each patient cost $750. Additional information can be found at www.stemlogix.com.

Umbilical Cord Blood–Derived Mesenchymal Stem Cells

EquStem (EquStem, Hackensack, NJ, USA) is the first commercial equine umbilical cord blood–derived stem cell bank in the United States. This company works in partnership with V-Care Biomedical GmbH (Leipzig, Germany) and the New Jersey Cord

Blood Bank/Eli Katz Umbilical Cord Blood Program at Community Blood Services (Allendale, NJ, USA) to provide isolation, expansion, and cryopreservation services for umbilical cord blood–derived MSCs. The goal is to preserve umbilical cord blood–derived MSCs for future sport horses to enable easy and rapid availability in case of injuries. The company also provides culture expansion of MSCs isolated from bone marrow aspirates.

EquStem provides training, supplies, and collection kits necessary to collect blood from the umbilical cord on foaling day or to harvest bone marrow from adult horses in the event of injury (www.equstem.com). After processing, isolation, and culture, umbilical cord blood–derived MSCs are cryogenically frozen and stored at −196°C for potential future therapeutic use. Alternatively, if bone marrow aspirates have been submitted for isolation and expansion, the processing technique and time period is fairly similar to those used by the other commercial laboratories described previously. To date there are no objective data addressing the clinical efficacy of umbilical cord blood–derived MSCs for musculoskeletal injuries.

Embryonic-Like Stem Cells

ESCs that have been previously isolated from horses and maintained in cell culture are an alternative therapeutic option to the currently available cell-based products. ESCs can potentially be used as allogenic or "off-the-shelf" cell sources to treat soft tissue injuries immediately after diagnosis. At present, Celavet (Celavet Inc, Oxnard, CA, USA) is the only company that has developed an equine ESC line (equine fetal-derived embryonic-like stem cells; OK 100) to treat tendon and ligament injuries. However, this cell-based therapy has not yet been approved by the US Food and Drug Administration (FDA) Center for Veterinary Medicine.

Nonetheless, preliminary data from an ongoing, multicenter (39 equine practices) study in the United States indicates that Celavet's fetal-derived ESCs are an effective therapy for acute and chronic tendinitis. In addition, promising results have been obtained at Cornell University in an experimental study determining the efficacy of fetal-derived ESCs for superficial digital flexor tendon repair.[34] At the present time, Celavet fetal-derived ESCs are at the investigational stage and undergoing further validation studies in qualified animal subjects under FDA guidelines. Although not currently available for general veterinary use, qualified veterinary practitioners can obtain and administer Celavet fetal-derived stem cells as participating investigators in Celavet's multicenter field studies. Additional information can be found at www.celavet.com.

SUMMARY

Equine practitioners have several cell-based therapeutic options available to treat musculoskeletal injuries in horses. Most of these therapies hold great potential as new treatment strategies for tendon and ligament injuries. However, the usefulness of these therapies to treat joint disease is unknown at this point. Despite promising results of experimental and clinical studies, clinical trials are still necessary to compare the safety and efficacy of current cell-based therapies with the current standard of care for musculoskeletal injuries in horses.

REFERENCES

1. Stocum DL. Regeneration of musculoskeletal tissues. In: Stocum DL, editor. Regenerative biology and medicine. Burlington (MA): Elsevier; 2006. p. 221–49.

2. Schnabel LV, Lynch ME, van der Meulen MC, et al. Mesenchymal stem cells and insulin-like growth factor-I gene-enhanced mesenchymal stem cells improve structural aspects of healing in equine flexor digitorum superficialis tendons. J Orthop Res 2009;27(10):1392-8.

3. Fortier LA, Potter HG, Rickey EJ, et al. Concentrated bone marrow aspirate improves full-thickness cartilage repair compared with microfracture in the equine model. J Bone Joint Surg Am 2010;92(10):1927-37.

4. Nixon AJ, Dahlgren LA, Haupt JL, et al. Effect of adipose-derived nucleated cell fractions on tendon repair in horses with collagenase-induced tendinitis. Am J Vet Res 2008;69(7):928-37.

5. Crovace A, Lacitignola L, Rossi G, et al. Histological and immunohistochemical evaluation of autologous cultured bone marrow mesenchymal stem cells and bone marrow mononucleated cells in collagenase-induced tendinitis of equine superficial digital flexor tendon. Vet Med Int 2010;2010. DOI: 10.4061/2010/250978.

6. Pacini S, Spinabella S, Trombi L, et al. Suspension of bone marrow-derived undifferentiated mesenchymal stromal cells for repair of superficial digital flexor tendon in race horses. Tissue Eng 2007;13(12):2949-55.

7. Smith RK. Mesenchymal stem cell therapy for equine tendinopathy. Disabil Rehabil 2008;30(20-22):1752-8.

8. Kisiday JD, Kopesky PW, Evans CH, et al. Evaluation of adult equine bone marrow- and adipose-derived progenitor cell chondrogenesis in hydrogel cultures. J Orthop Res 2008;26(3):322-31.

9. Toupadakis CA, Wong A, Genetos DC, et al. Comparison of the osteogenic potential of equine mesenchymal stem cells from bone marrow, adipose tissue, umbilical cord blood, and umbilical cord tissue. Am J Vet Res 2010;71(10):1237-45.

10. Braun J, Hack A, Weis-Klemm M, et al. Evaluation of the osteogenic and chondrogenic differentiation capacities of equine adipose tissue-derived mesenchymal stem cells. Am J Vet Res 2010;71(10):1228-36.

11. Vidal MA, Robinson SO, Lopez MJ, et al. Comparison of chondrogenic potential in equine mesenchymal stromal cells derived from adipose tissue and bone marrow. Vet Surg 2008;37(8):713-24.

12. Fortier LA, Nixon AJ, Williams J, et al. Isolation and chondrocytic differentiation of equine bone marrow-derived mesenchymal stem cells. Am J Vet Res 1998;59(9):1182-7.

13. Giovannini S, Brehm W, Mainil-Varlet P, et al. Multilineage differentiation potential of equine blood-derived fibroblast-like cells. Differentiation 2008;76(2):118-29.

14. Colleoni S, Bottani E, Tessaro I, et al. Isolation, growth and differentiation of equine mesenchymal stem cells: effect of donor, source, amount of tissue and supplementation with basic fibroblast growth factor. Vet Res Commun 2009;33(8):811-21.

15. Vidal MA, Kilroy GE, Lopez MJ, et al. Characterization of equine adipose tissue-derived stromal cells: adipogenic and osteogenic capacity and comparison with bone marrow-derived mesenchymal stromal cells. Vet Surg 2007;36(7):613-22.

16. Guest DJ, Smith MR, Allen WR. Monitoring the fate of autologous and allogeneic mesenchymal progenitor cells injected into the superficial digital flexor tendon of horses: preliminary study. Equine Vet J 2008;40(2):178-81.

17. Guest DJ, Smith MR, Allen WR. Equine embryonic stem-like cells and mesenchymal stromal cells have different survival rates and migration patterns following their injection into damaged superficial digital flexor tendon. Equine Vet J 2010;42(7):636-42.

18. Frisbie DD, Kisiday JD, Kawcak CE, et al. Evaluation of adipose-derived stromal vascular fraction or bone marrow-derived mesenchymal stem cells for treatment of osteoarthritis. J Orthop Res 2009;27(12):1675–80.
19. Bourzac C, Smith LC, Vincent P, et al. Isolation of equine bone marrow-derived mesenchymal stem cells: a comparison between three protocols. Equine Vet J 2010;42(6):519–27.
20. Ferris D, Frisbie D, Kisiday J, et al. Clinical evaluation of bone marrow-derived mesenchymal stem cells in naturally occurring joint disease. Regen Med 2009; 4(6):S16.
21. Ferris DJ, Frisbie DD, Kisiday JD, et al. Clinical follow up of horses treated with bone marrow derived mesenchymal stem cells for musculoskeletal lesions. Proc AAEP 2009;55:59–60.
22. Smith RK. Results of treatment of bone marrow derived mesenchymal stem cell therapy. Proc WVOC 2010;3:248–9.
23. Thoesen MS, Berg-Foels WS, Stokol T, et al. Use of a centrifugation-based, point-of-care device for production of canine autologous bone marrow and platelet concentrates. Am J Vet Res 2006;67(10):1655–61.
24. Fortier LA, Smith RK. Regenerative medicine for tendinous and ligamentous injuries of sport horses. Vet Clin North Am Equine Pract 2008;24(1):191–201.
25. Yoshioka T, Mishima H, Akaogi H, et al. Concentrated autologous bone marrow aspirate transplantation treatment for corticosteroid-induced osteonecrosis of the femoral head in systemic lupus erythematosus. Int Orthop 2010. DOI: 10.1007/s00264-010-1048-y.
26. Jager M, Herten M, Fochtmann U, et al. Bridging the gap: bone marrow aspiration concentrate reduces autologous bone grafting in osseous defects. J Orthop Res 2011;29(2):173–80.
27. Di Bella C, Dozza B, Frisoni T, et al. Injection of demineralized bone matrix with bone marrow concentrate improves healing in unicameral bone cyst. Clin Orthop Relat Res 2010;468(11):3047–55.
28. Hernigou P, Poignard A, Beaujean F, et al. Percutaneous autologous bone-marrow grafting for nonunions. Influence of the number and concentration of progenitor cells. J Bone Joint Surg Am 2005;87(7):1430–7.
29. Bell R, Snyder J, Buerchler S, et al. Intralesional injection of regenerative medicine products as a treatment for tendonitis of the deep digital flexor tendon in the equine distal extremity. Proc Eur Coll Vet Surg 2010;19:68.
30. Dyson SJ, Murray R, Schramme MC. Lameness associated with foot pain: results of magnetic resonance imaging in 199 horses (January 2001–December 2003) and response to treatment. Equine Vet J 2005;37(2):113–21.
31. Frisbie DD, Smith RK. Clinical update on the use of mesenchymal stem cells in equine orthopaedics. Equine Vet J 2010;42(1):86–9.
32. Harman RJ, Cowles B, Orava C, et al. A retrospective review of 52 cases of suspensory ligament injury in sport horses treated with adipose-derived stem and regenerative cell therapy. Proc Vet Orthop Soc 2007;34:28.
33. Leppänen M, Heikkilä P, Katiskalahti T, et al. Follow-up of recovery of equine tendon and ligament injuries 18–24 months after treatment with enriched autologous adipose-derived mesenchymal stem cells: a clinical study. Regen Med 2009;4(6):S21–2.
34. Watts AE, Yeager A, Kopyov OV, et al. Fetal-derived embryonic-like stem cells improve healing in a large animal flexor tendonitis model. Stem Cell Res Ther 2011;2(1):4.

Evidence-Based Medicine and Stem Cell Therapy: How Do We Know Such Technologies are Safe and Efficacious?

Peter D. Clegg, MA, Vet MB, PhD[a],*, Gina L. Pinchbeck, BVSc, PhD[b]

KEYWORDS

• Stem cell • Evidence-based medicine • Horse

The introduction of stem cell therapies provides huge opportunities to the veterinary profession. Stem cell therapy offers potential solutions for a variety of difficult chronic diseases for which current pharmacologic or surgical approaches often do not provide truly efficacious treatments. Furthermore, such cell-based therapies currently are being introduced within a liberal legal and regulatory environment, which means that such therapies can be rapidly translated from research laboratory settings to mainstream clinical practice.

However, with the many opportunities that come with cell-based therapies, there are risks and dangers potentially lying in wait for advocates of such new technologies. Many of the conditions that seem ideally suited for stem cell treatment have had a long history of introduction of revolutionary treatments that have subsequently been shown to be either not efficacious or even deleterious for the animal's recovery. Injuries to the superficial digital flexor tendon are a prime example of an injury for which there is a strong clinical need to develop novel therapeutic options, although historically novel therapies have ultimately lacked efficacy.[1] Furthermore, the often rapid commercialization of cell-based therapies, although allowing easy access to these treatments for the veterinary profession, has some danger of unsubstantiated claims being promulgated to both veterinarians and the equine industry.

The authors have nothing to disclose.
[a] Department of Musculoskeletal Biology, University of Liverpool, Leahurst Campus, Chester High Road, Neston, Cheshire, CH64 7TE, UK
[b] Department of Epidemiology, University of Liverpool, Leahurst Campus, Chester High Road, Neston, Cheshire, CH64 7TE, UK
* Corresponding author.
E-mail address: p.d.clegg@liverpool.ac.uk

Vet Clin Equine 27 (2011) 373–382
doi:10.1016/j.cveq.2011.04.002
0749-0739/11/$ – see front matter © 2011 Elsevier Inc. All rights reserved.

It is imperative that an evidence-based approach is taken during the development of cell-based therapies, with the best quality evidence being sought to determine the true efficacy of such approaches. The current clinical literature relating to cell-based therapies frequently relies on study designs that do not provide robust evidence of benefit. The challenge for the future is to design and develop studies that do provide acceptable evidence for the role of such therapies in equine medicine. This challenge will have to be achieved in an environment in which the gold standard of evidence-based medicine (EBM) (the blinded randomized control trial) is always going to be difficult to undertake in equine veterinary science because of the expense of running such a study in an ethical manner, that is appropriately controlled, is of sufficient power, and has appropriate outcome measures.

EBM

The term EBM was first published scientifically in 1992, with the term defined in 1996 using a definition that is still widely used today: "The conscientious, explicit and judicious use of current best evidence about individual patient care."[2] The practice of EBM allows the integration of an individual's clinical expertise with the best available evidence from systematic research, specifically incorporating the best information from clinical research and the best clinical judgment of the clinician.[3]

The key to EBM is the requirement for clinicians to be familiar with the types of evidence that are available to them and, in particular, to be able to determine the strengths and weaknesses inherent in the differing types of evidence.[3] A system of ranking sources of evidence into a hierarchy based on their relative strengths has developed, which has frequently led to the establishment of evidence pyramids to illustrate the hierarchical nature of different forms of evidence.[4] Several methodologies have been proposed for distinguishing studies that provide differing levels of evidence. In the United Kingdom National Health Service, historically, a 4-level method of distinguishing evidence has been applied, based on ideas developed by the Oxford Centre for Evidence-Based Medicine, as follows:

1. Class A studies generate the highest quality evidence, relying on data produced from high-quality, double-blinded, placebo-controlled clinical trials.
2. Class B evidence is derived from high-quality clinical trials that use historical controls.
3. Class C evidence is obtained from uncontrolled case series.
4. Class D studies generate the least informative data, derived from anecdotal clinical reports or expert clinical appraisal or extrapolated from in vitro or other benchtop experiments.

More recently, this hierarchy has been further adapted into a more complex 5-step hierarchy.[5] In North America, a 4- or 5-level hierarchy for ranking the quality of evidence is commonly used.[3,4]

A recent adaptation of this system has been used in veterinary medicine, reviewing the efficacy of therapies for canine osteoarthritis.[6] This approach uses a ranking system produced by the US Food and Drug Administration (FDA), based on work by the American Dietetic Association.[7] This system uses an approach that ranks studies by 6 criteria.

1. The design of the study: type I studies are randomized, controlled, interventional studies; type II studies are prospective, observational, cohort studies; type III studies are nonrandomized interventions using either concurrent or historical

controls, case-control studies, or experimental data; and type IV studies are either cross-sectional studies or involve analysis of secondary end points in either intervention trials or case series
2. The scientific quality of studies
3. The quality of the data provided by the studies
4. The consistency of results of the studies
5. The relevance of the study to the reduction of the risk of the particular disease or condition under investigation; this is a measure of how applicable the findings are on a physiologic basis
6. The study's level of comfort: this phrase is used to convey the overall strength of the evidence and is divided into studies that exhibit high, moderate, low, or extremely low levels of comfort. High level of comfort studies are defined as high-quality type I or II designs that incorporate sufficient animals and provide results that are relevant to the target population. Extremely low level of comfort studies are type III studies of moderate to low quality, with insufficient animals for a conclusive result to be reached. In such studies, results can be extrapolated to the target population with only a low degree of confidence.[6]

Differing methods of evidence evaluation can produce differing conclusions regarding the quality of evidence within a publication. This finding has been recognized in assessments of studies on canine osteoarthritis in which 2 differing systematic reviews[6,8] produced conflicting opinions on a randomized controlled study using a specific therapeutic agent in canine osteoarthritis.[9] The initial systematic review identified this study to be of high quality,[8] whereas the subsequent review determined that this study provided little evidence that the therapy would have physiologically meaningful and achievable effects.[6] The methodology used in the latter systematic review emphasized the importance of high-quality study designs that are both randomized and placebo controlled and have readily identifiable primary outcome variables as well as the means to assess these objectively.[6]

One of the major issues facing many aspects of equine veterinary clinical practice is the lack of appropriate rigorously controlled clinical studies that can serve as the basis for systematic reviews and meta-analyses. The current equine scientific literature is not sufficiently large or of an appropriate quality to support such meta-analyses. However, it will be increasingly important that studies designed to demonstrate clinical efficacy of cell-based therapies adopt study designs that provide the highest quality evidence.

CURRENT EVIDENCE-BASED STUDIES IN EQUINE STEM CELL THERAPY

The concept of stem cell therapy has been advocated for more than 10 years, and, in human medicine, there have been a growing number of clinical reports of increasing quality, documenting the use of stem cell therapies, particularly relating to myocardial infarction.[10–12] Furthermore, clinical studies have been published relating to the use of mesenchymal stem cells in other conditions, for example, therapy for skin repair in diabetes[13] and therapy for Crohn disease.[14] Despite such evidence-based approaches being adopted, there have often been concerns that such cell-based therapies may be the subject of exaggerated claims.[15–17] In human orthopedic applications, there are currently few high-quality clinical trials that address the efficacy of stem cell therapies in a clinical setting,[18] although there are several clinical trials underway investigating specific questions relating to cell therapy efficacy, particularly relating to cartilage repair.

In the horse, most published clinical studies address the use of stem cell therapies in the treatment of tendon and ligament injuries. This literature includes several experimental studies that use the collagenase model of tendonitis to model tendon strain pathology. Many of these studies are controlled but often lack sufficient experimental power because of the common problem of sample size limitations in horse-based studies. Furthermore, the issue of power is frequently compounded by considerable interanimal variability of pathologic conditions, which is often seen in the collagenase model of tendinitis. Accepting these observations, such experimental studies can provide valuable insights into approaches that can be taken forward into clinical studies. Examples of such studies include the use of adipose-derived cells,[19] bone marrow–derived cells,[20,21] bone marrow–derived cells transfected with growth factors,[22] and embryonic-derived cells.[23] Other models have been used to investigate cell survival and immunogenicity within tendons.[24,25]

There are an increasing number of publications describing case series of naturally occurring tendon and ligament injuries in client-owned horses treated with stem cells.[21,26–29] Such studies do contain interesting data, provide information on relevant techniques and approaches, and identify a lack of detectable adverse effects. However, the quality of the evidence generated by these studies is inherently weak because of their lack of randomization and blinding and the use of historical control populations for comparisons. Furthermore, the outcome parameters being measured as success vary between studies and can lack objectivity. The use of historical control data to act as a comparison for outcomes can be an issue in comparing the results of treatment of tendon diseases and is likely to lead to considerable bias. The healing of the tendon injury is likely to be greatly influenced by the management of the animal in the rehabilitation phase and, in particular, how the return to exercise is managed and monitored. It is highly probable that the healing response of a horse that is managed simply by pasture turnout and is rapidly returned to fast work differs from that of a horse subjected to a highly structured period of box rest and controlled exercise that is monitored and staged in the context of serial ultrasound examinations. Furthermore, client-owned horses that have undergone costly cell therapy treatments may be managed more closely than an animal for which there has been little investment in expensive therapy. Horses that are destined for different competitive disciplines have different outcomes for the same injury. Thus, care has to be taken in assessing outcome comparisons based on historical controls that are not always matched to the use of the target horse population and, in particular, do not control for variations in the all-important postinjury rehabilitation period.

In the treatment of joint disease, there are several important experimental studies that inform the use of mesenchymal stem cell therapy in the horse,[30,31] although there are currently no published studies that provide evidence for joint therapy using mesenchymal stem cells in clinical patients. There are several ongoing studies detailing the clinical use of such therapies for joint disease that are likely to provide valuable evidence in the near future.

OUTCOME MEASURES IN EQUINE STEM CELL THERAPY

The use of appropriate and robust outcomes that can be objectively assessed is critical to successful EBM. Furthermore, such measures should relate to the eventual clinical outcomes rather than some biochemical or imaging measurement that may not have a defined physiologic relationship and may only have an indirect association to functional recovery. Furthermore, outcome measures that can be obtained in vivo are hugely advantageous because this allows development of longitudinal studies, which have both ethical and practical advantages.

Tendons and Ligaments

Several clinical, biochemical, transcriptional, mechanical, and ultrastructural outcome measures have been used to determine the response to cell-based therapies.

In vivo measures

The 2 most common outcome measures for successful treatment of tendon and ligament injury are percentage return to previous level of activity and reinjury rate once the horse is back in full activity.[21,26,29] Often such publications use a key reference[32] to compare these outcome measures with historical controls. Imaging methodologies, particularly ultrasonography, are widely used.[22,27,29] Although ultrasonography can be used semiquantitatively to measure the cross-sectional areas of the tendon and lesion, echogenicity, and fiber pattern linearity, these measures frequently carry some degree of subjectivity. Furthermore, the sensitivity of the technique has to be questioned because a study has concluded that there is a benefit to cellular therapy, even though there has been no demonstrable improvement in the ultrasound parameters.[22] Furthermore, it has not been convincingly shown that specific alterations in ultrasound imaging parameters demonstrably alter the prognosis and eventual outcome. Recent advances and access to magnetic resonance imaging (MRI) technologies have made such approaches applicable to assessing cell-based therapies in the horse.[23] The development of standing MRI facilitates longitudinal clinical studies in horses; standing MRI provides the great advantage of avoiding the need for examinations under general anesthesia.[33]

Kinematics and force plate analyses of horse gait and locomotion have been used widely in equine musculoskeletal research for several years but, to date, have rarely been applied in determining the response to cell-based therapies for tendon diseases in the horse.[34,35] Recently, a biomechanical approach to determine tendon mechanics in vivo has been specifically developed to identify response to tendon therapies.[36] Although such an approach requires validation in a therapeutic setting, it would seem to have considerable potential.

Postmortem studies

The examination of a tendon tissue at postmortem can be a powerful tool to assess therapeutic benefit, although there may not be a definitive physiologic link between defining a specific parameter in a tendon tissue and any eventual clinical outcome. This is probably most apparent in measuring matrix components or gene expression profiles within tendon tissues at specific time points after injury. It remains to be resolved whether alterations in levels or distribution of a specific factor (gene or protein) within tissue are linked to a better or worse clinical outcome. A variety of gene transcripts and proteins are commonly measured in tendon stem cell studies, in particular, collagen types I and III, cartilage oligomeric matrix protein and a variety of growth factors, and proteinases. Cellularity can be estimated by measuring the DNA concentration, whereas fibrochondrogenic differentiation is often determined by glycosaminoglycan accumulation. Gross postmortem appearance and size of the tendon can also be assessed. Histologic organization of the tendon matrix is a common postmortem determinant and can be scored to provide an objective measure,[19] and although these assessments can provide powerful information on matrix organization that is likely to be correlated with better clinical outcomes, no causal relationship between specific histologic parameters and clinical outcome has yet been established. Both destructive and nondestructive mechanical testing of the tendon tissue in vitro is frequently performed and can give important information on the mechanical and material properties of the tendon after differing therapies. Biomechanical assessments generally involve single, progressive, tensile loading testing as opposed to the high-frequency, submaximal, repetitive loading that tendons are subject to in vivo.

The major limitation of postmortem analysis is that the data are generally cross-sectional, and it is expensive to obtain the specimens, especially when multiple time points are investigated. Furthermore, because of the considerable variability in the current experimental disease models and in naturally occurring disease, the data produced are often noisy and inconsistent. The horse is genetically heterogeneous, and it is also not always possible to fully standardize the post-therapy protocols with respect to movement and exercise. These issues frequently result in studies that lack power, particularly because sample sizes are often small due to cost and ethical considerations.

Research needs to develop methodologies to provide better evidence in the live horse, and it is likely that the use of both advanced imaging methodologies and in vivo mechanical testing is fundamental to the development of a strong evidence-based approach for the investigations of cell-based therapies in the horse.

Joint and Cartilage Studies

For determining outcome measures relating to joints, many of the issues relating to tendons are relevant. Again one of the major concerns is whether the entities being measured are relevant to the ultimate clinical outcome.

In vivo measures

Although biomechanical and kinematic studies are available to determine joint motion and loading, study outcomes are frequently limited to semiobjective quantification of lameness scores.[30] Imaging is a potentially powerful tool for determining cartilage repair in vivo. Second-look arthroscopy can be used to examine and objectively score sites of cartilage repair.[31] Furthermore, such approaches allow for both biopsy of osteochondral tissue from the repair site and some assessment of the mechanical properties of repair tissue using arthroscopic indentation.[37] MRI can be used for noninvasive cartilage assessment in vivo, although a high-field (up to 3 T) magnet is required to fully define cartilage structure and integrity. This requirement precludes the use of standing MRI; to date, studies have relied on the imaging of small ponies under general anesthesia or on cross-sectional imaging of postmortem specimens.[38] MRI quantification of cartilage matrix components can be enhanced by the use of specific contrast agents, for instance, gadolinium.[38,39] Fluid biomarkers offer potential in defining aspects of cartilage repair and joint health, although currently such approaches seem to have distinct limitations.[40,41]

Postmortem studies

As with the assessment of tendon healing, a wide variety of measures have been used to assess outcomes for cartilage repair and joint health in postmortem specimens. There is a much wider acceptance and validation of histologic assessment as an outcome measure in joints, although there is still some concern that a defined link between a specific score and clinical outcome is lacking.[42,43] Mechanical testing of cartilage can give some indication of the quality of repair.[44,45] Measurement and localization of specific proteins and gene transcripts, most commonly relating to chondrogenesis, are frequently performed.[31] Although providing some indication of the degree of chondrogenic or fibrochondrogenic differentiation, these analyses may not always provide a direct relationship with clinical outcome.

SUMMARY

The use of cell-based therapies for orthopedic repair in the horse has considerable clinical support. The evidence base for clinical efficacy at the moment is not strong, although there is a growing body of lower-level evidence that both supports continuing clinical investigation and currently does not identify particularly adverse effects associated with its use. What is now required is the development of more robust clinical evidence to fully determine efficacy and appropriate therapeutic applications; this is going to be challenging for the equine veterinary profession. There are few examples of successful high-quality clinical trials in the horse, and, where they have been performed, they have often been complex and expensive to perform. The ability to randomize treatments and blind investigators to the treatments has often been unsuccessful, with the industry often reluctant to accept randomization in experimental design. The costs of such trials can be large, and in a world in which the horse is often seen as a low research priority, it is hard to see how such investigations leading to best evidence will be funded.

Consensus is required on what are the most appropriate outcome measures to define success. Resources should be put into developing such outcome measures that are robust and appropriate and, in particular, allow studies to be performed non-invasively in client-owned horses. The ability to perform longitudinal studies in clinical populations will be key to obtaining a robust evidence base for validation of such technologies. Undoubtedly, there will still be a place for experimental horse studies to address specific questions that can be best answered using appropriate experimental models. The development of appropriate and clinically relevant experimental disease models to investigate orthopedic repair are required.[46] The use of cell-based therapy in the treatment of equine injury has immense potential, and it is important that strong evidence to support its benefits is now obtained.

REFERENCES

1. Vaughan LC, Edwards GB, Gerring EL. Tendon injuries in horses treated with carbon fibre implants. Equine Vet J 1985;17:45–50.
2. Sackett DL, Rosenberg WM, Gray JA, et al. Evidence based medicine: what it is and what it isn't. BMJ 1996;312:71–2.
3. Holmes MA, Ramey DA. An introduction to evidence-based veterinary medicine. Vet Clin North Am Equine Pract 2007;23(2):191–200.
4. Aragon CL, Budsberg SC. Applications of evidence-based medicine: cranial cruciate ligament injury repair in the dog. Vet Surg 2005;34:93–8.
5. OCEBM Levels of Evidence Working Group. The Oxford 2011 levels of evidence (Oxford Centre for Evidence-Based Medicine). 2011. Available at: http://www.cebm.net/mod_product/design/files/CEBM-Levels-of-Evidence-2.1.pdf. Accessed 29 May, 2011.
6. Sanderson RO, Beata C, Flipo RM, et al. Systematic review of the management of canine osteoarthritis. Vet Rec 2009;164:418–24.
7. Myers EF, Pritchett E, Johnson EQ. Evidence-based practice guides vs. protocols: what's the difference? J Am Diet Assoc 2001;101:1085–90.
8. Aragon CL, Hofmeister EH, Budsberg SC. Systematic review of clinical trials of treatments for osteoarthritis in dogs. J Am Vet Med Assoc 2007;230:514–21.

9. Innes JF, Fuller CJ, Grover ER, et al. Randomised, double-blind, placebo-controlled parallel group study of P54FP for the treatment of dogs with osteoarthritis. Vet Rec 2003;152:457–60.

10. Davis DR, Stewart DJ. Autologous cell therapy for cardiac repair. Expert Opin Biol Ther 2011;11:489–508.

11. Hare JM, Traverse JH, Henry TD, et al. A randomized, double-blind, placebo-controlled, dose-escalation study of intravenous adult human mesenchymal stem cells (prochymal) after acute myocardial infarction. J Am Coll Cardiol 2009;54:2277–86.

12. Wollert KC, Meyer GP, Lotz J, et al. Intracoronary autologous bone-marrow cell transfer after myocardial infarction: the BOOST randomised controlled clinical trial. Lancet 2004;364:141–8.

13. Lu D, Chen B, Liang Z, et al. Comparison of bone marrow mesenchymal stem cells with bone marrow-derivedmononuclear cells for treatment of diabetic critical limb ischemia and foot ulcer: a double-blind, randomized, controlled trial. Diabetes Res Clin Pract 2011;92:26–36.

14. Duijvestein M, Vos AC, Roelofs H, et al. Autologous bone marrow-derived mesenchymal stromal cell treatment for refractory luminal Crohn's disease: results of a phase I study. Gut 2010;59:1662–9.

15. Braude P, Minger SL, Warwick RM. Stem cell therapy: hope or hype? BMJ 2005; 330:1159–60.

16. Nadig RR. Stem cell therapy - hype or hope? a review. J Conserv Dent 2009;12: 131–8.

17. Scolding N. Stem-cell therapy: hope and hype. Lancet 2005;365:2073–5.

18. Wakitani S, Okabe T, Horibe S, et al. Safety of autologous bone marrow-derived mesenchymal stem cell transplantation for cartilage repair in 41 patients with 45 joints followed for up to 11 years and 5 months. J Tissue Eng Regen Med 2011;5:146–50.

19. Nixon AJ, Dahlgren LA, Haupt JL, et al. Effect of adipose-derived nucleated cell fractions on tendon repair in horses with collagenase-induced tendinitis. Am J Vet Res 2008;69:928–37.

20. Crovace A, Lacitignola L, De Siena R, et al. Cell therapy for tendon repair in horses: an experimental study. Vet Res Commun 2007;31(Suppl 1):281–3.

21. Lacitignola L, Crovace A, Rossi G, et al. Cell therapy for tendinitis, experimental and clinical report. Vet Res Commun 2008;32(Suppl 1):S33–8.

22. Schnabel LV, Lynch ME, van der Meulen MC, et al. Mesenchymal stem cells and insulin-like growth factor-I gene-enhanced mesenchymal stem cells improve structural aspects of healing in equine flexor digitorum superficialis tendons. J Orthop Res 2009;27:1392–8.

23. Watts AE, Yeager AE, Kopyov OV, et al. Fetal derived embryonic-like stem cells improve healing in a large animal flexor tendonitis model. Stem Cell Res Ther 2011;2(1):4.

24. Guest DJ, Smith MR, Allen WR. Monitoring the fate of autologous and allogeneic mesenchymal progenitor cells injected into the superficial digital flexor tendon of horses: preliminary study. Equine Vet J 2008;40:178–81.

25. Guest DJ, Smith MR, Allen WR. Equine embryonic stem-like cells and mesenchymal stromal cells have different survival rates and migration patterns following their injection into damaged superficial digital flexor tendon. Equine Vet J 2010; 42:636–42.

26. Burk J, Brehm W. Stem cell therapy of tendon injuries—clinical outcome in 98 cases. PFERDEHEILKUNDE 2011;27(2):153.

27. Pacini S, Spinabella S, Trombi L, et al. Suspension of bone marrow-derived undifferentiated mesenchymal stromal cells for repair of superficial digital flexor tendon in race horses. Tissue Eng 2007;13:2949–55.
28. Richardson LE, Dudhia J, Clegg PD, et al. Stem cells in veterinary medicine—attempts at regenerating equine tendon after injury. Trends Biotechnol 2007;25:409–16.
29. Smith RK. Mesenchymal stem cell therapy for equine tendinopathy. Disabil Rehabil 2008;30:1752–8.
30. Frisbie DD, Kisiday JD, Kawcak CE, et al. Evaluation of adipose-derived stromal vascular fraction or bone marrow-derived mesenchymal stem cells for treatment of osteoarthritis. J Orthop Res 2009;27:1675–80.
31. Wilke MM, Nydam DV, Nixon AJ. Enhanced early chondrogenesis in articular defects following arthroscopic mesenchymal stem cell implantation in an equine model. J Orthop Res 2007;25:913–25.
32. Dyson SJ. Medical management of superficial digital flexor tendonitis: a comparative study in 219 horses (1992–2000). Equine Vet J 2004;36:415–9.
33. Milner P, Sidwell S, Talbot A, et al. Short term temporal alterations in MR signal in primary lesions identified in the deep digital flexor tendon of the equine digit. Equine Vet J 2011, in press.
34. Clayton HM, Schamhardt HC, Willemen MA, et al. Kinematics and ground reaction forces in horses with superficial digital flexor tendinitis. Am J Vet Res 2000;61:191–6.
35. Clayton HM, Schamhardt HC, Willemen MA, et al. Net joint moments and joint powers in horses with superficial digital flexor tendinitis. Am J Vet Res 2000;61:197–201.
36. Dakin S, Jespers K, Warner S, et al. The relationship between in vivo limb and in vitro tendon mechanics after injury: a potential novel clinical tool for monitoring tendon repair. Equine Vet J 2011, in press. DOI: 10.1111/j.2042-3306.2010.00303.x.
37. Toyras J, Lyyra-Laitinen T, Niinimaki M, et al. Estimation of the Young's modulus of articular cartilage using an arthroscopic indentation instrument and ultrasonic measurement of tissue thickness. J Biomech 2001;34:251–6.
38. Fortier LA, Potter HG, Rickey EJ, et al. Concentrated bone marrow aspirate improves full-thickness cartilage repair compared with microfracture in the equine model. J Bone Joint Surg Am 2010;92:1927–37.
39. Bashir A, Gray ML, Boutin RD, et al. Glycosaminoglycan in articular cartilage: in vivo assessment with delayed Gd(DTPA)(2-)-enhanced MR imaging. Radiology 1997;205:551–8.
40. Garvican ER, Vaughan-Thomas A, Innes JF, et al. Biomarkers of cartilage turnover. Part 1: markers of collagen degradation and synthesis. Vet J 2010;185:36–42.
41. Garvican ER, Vaughan-Thomas A, Clegg PD, et al. Biomarkers of cartilage turnover. Part 2: non-collagenous markers. Vet J 2010;185:43–9.
42. Aigner T, Cook JL, Gerwin N, et al. Histopathology atlas of animal model systems—overview of guiding principles. Osteoarthritis Cartilage 2010;18(Suppl 3):S2–6.
43. McIlwraith CW, Frisbie DD, Kawcak CE, et al. The OARSI histopathology initiative—recommendations for histological assessments of osteoarthritis in the horse. Osteoarthritis Cartilage 2010;18(Suppl 3):S93–105.
44. Jin H, Lewis JL. Determination of Poisson's ratio of articular cartilage by indentation using different-sized indenters. J Biomech Eng 2004;126:138–45.

45. Kiviranta P, Rieppo J, Korhonen RK, et al. Collagen network primarily controls Poisson's ratio of bovine articular cartilage in compression. J Orthop Res 2006; 24:690–9.
46. Schramme M, Hunter S, Campbell N, et al. A surgical tendonitis model in horses: technique, clinical, ultrasonographic and histological characterisation. Vet Comp Orthop Traumatol 2010;23:231–9.

The Regulation of Veterinary Regenerative Medicine and the Potential Impact of Such Regulation on Clinicians and Firms Commercializing These Treatments

Karl M. Nobert, Esq

KEYWORDS

- Veterinary • Regenerative medicine • FDA • Law • Drug
- Labeling • Misbranding • Regenerative services

The practice of veterinary medicine, including regenerative medicine, falls under the regulatory jurisdiction of the American Veterinary Medical Association, although the products used in that practice squarely fall under the US Food and Drug Administration's (FDA or the agency) regulatory authority. This article provides the reader with an overview of the FDA's regulation of animal products generally; its regulation of veterinary regenerative medicine specifically, including products, such as stem cell therapy and platelet-rich plasma; the potential impact on practicing veterinarians; and the possible impact of the FDA's rules on the commercialization of such products. It is the author's hope that the included discussion provides a comprehensible overview of the federal regulation of veterinary regenerative medicine and the products used in the practice and helps to mitigate the regulatory risks associated with the marketing and promotion of such marketed therapies and products in the United States.

The author has nothing to disclose.
K&L Gates LLP, 1601 K Street, NW, Washington, DC 20006, USA
E-mail address: karl.nobert@klgates.com

Vet Clin Equine 27 (2011) 383–391
doi:10.1016/j.cveq.2011.06.002
0749-0739/11/$ – see front matter © 2011 Published by Elsevier Inc.

OVERVIEW

A veterinary product's regulatory status is judged by its composition and intended use. Intended use is determined by a product's label and any accompanying promotional materials, such as brochures, detailers, Web sites, articles, trade show materials, television and radio advertisements, and consumer testimonials. Deemed labeling generally, the FDA requires all such materials to be truthful and not misleading. False and misleading labeling renders a product misbranded and subject to potential FDA enforcement action.

Veterinary regenerative medicine is a new product concept to the FDA in terms of regulation. Historically, veterinary products, such as blood, plasma, and tissues, have been regulated as simply biologics or as animal drug products by either the FDA's Center of Veterinary Medicine (CVM) under the Federal Food, Drug, and Cosmetic Act (FDCA) or the US Department of Agriculture's Center for Veterinary Biologics under the Public Health Service Act, or some combination of both. Today, all indications suggest that the FDA is asserting primary and exclusive regulatory authority over veterinary regenerative therapies and products, and intends to treat them as drugs for regulatory purposes (with limited exceptions), requiring prior review and approval. Specific regulatory requirements and guidance covering the practice have yet to be published by the FDA, as has been done for human cellular and tissue products. At the time of writing this article, there are no FDA-approved veterinary cellular or tissue products on the market, much less approved products specifically intended for use in the practice of regenerative medicine. There are suggestions, however, that there are currently several such products undergoing FDA review. No indication has been given regarding when these products might be approved for marketing and sales.

Designation as a new animal drug product raises significant regulatory responsibilities and concerns for a firm or individual seeking to commercialize a product. Although some regulatory cover is provided to academics and investigators using cell- and tissue-derived products for research in a university or similar laboratory-type setting, designation as a new animal drug product by the FDA will have a significant impact on the veterinary regenerative medicine industry as a whole and at least some yet-to-be-determined impact on clinicians who prescribe and treat their patients with regenerative medicine.

AN INTRODUCTION TO THE REGULATION OF VETERINARY DRUG PRODUCTS IN THE UNITED STATES

All indications suggest that until the FDA adopts specific regulations or guidelines, veterinary regenerative medicine will be governed under CVM's existing statutory and regulatory framework for veterinary drug products, with heavy reliance on the rules covering human cellular- and tissue-based products. Thus, to understand how veterinary regenerative medicine might be regulated in the future, it is important to understand how CVM currently regulates approved animal drug products.

The FDA regulates the drugs that veterinarians use to treat animals, including biologics, pursuant to the FDCA and its implementing regulations at 21 CFR Parts 510 to 514. A product intended for veterinary use can be regulated as a feed, drug, or biologic or medical device. In the case of veterinary regenerative medicine, the definitions of a new animal drug and a biologic are particularly important. A new animal drug is a drug "intended for use in animals, other than man, ... [that is] not generally recognized, among experts qualified by scientific training and experience to evaluate the safety and effectiveness of animal drugs, as safe and effective for use under the conditions prescribed, recommended, or suggested in the labeling."[1] FDA review and approval is required before a new animal drug product may be marketed and sold in the United States.[2] Alternatively, veterinary biologics include vaccines, bacterins, diagnostics, and other items that are used to prevent, treat, or diagnose animal diseases and that "generally work through some immunologic method or process."[3,4]

Product classification and, by extension, regulation depends on a variety of factors, including mode of action, intended use, and labeling. The FDA has indicated that animal cellular- and tissue-based products will most likely be treated as new animal drug products requiring agency review and approval. It has been suggested that such designation is appropriate based on the definition of biologic and the fact that regenerative products generally do not work through an immunologic method or process.

The FDA new drug review and approval process entails establishing that a proposed product is safe and effective for its intended use. The concept of safety encompasses the safety of the animal itself, the safety of the persons administering the drug or otherwise associated with the animal, the safety of any food products derived from the animal, and the drug's impact on the environment.[5] Effectiveness, however, means that the product will consistently and uniformly do what the labeling claims. It is traditionally shown through appropriately constructed models and other testing.

Before testing of the investigational product can begin, an Investigational New Animal Drug Application (INADA) will need to be opened. An INADA allows a manufacturer to ship an unapproved new animal drug product in interstate commerce for the purpose of conducting research to collect data needed to support the safety and efficacy of the proposed drug product. The collected safety and efficacy data is then assembled and submitted to the FDA in the form of a New Animal Drug Application (NADA) for review and possible approval.

CVM recommends contacting the agency early in the process to discuss a proposed product and its potential regulatory designation, the approval process generally, and the types of studies that might be needed to support an application.

FDA's REGULATION OF HUMAN REGENERATIVE MEDICINE

In April 2006, the FDA issued regulations specific to cellular and tissue-based products, including stem cells, for human use. In some cases, cellular products are treated as drug products under these regulations. Alternatively, they treated simply as biologics. Because of the similarities in the mode of action of these products and that of their animal counterparts, one can look to the FDA's regulation of human cellular- and tissue-based therapies and products for guidance on how similar veterinary products might be regulated.

Cellular- and tissue-based therapies and products intended for therapeutic purposes in humans are regulated as human cells, tissues, and cellular- and tissue-based products (HCT/Ps).[6] HCT/Ps are defined as "articles containing or consisting of human cells or tissues that are intended for implantation, transplantation, infusion, or transfer into a human recipient."[7] Examples include bone, ligament, skin, dura mater, stem cells, cartilage cells, and various other cellular- and tissue-based products. A distinction is made between unprocessed source material and processed material with a more rigorous level of regulatory scrutiny being applied to the latter. Discussed in the HCT/P regulations, such scrutiny covers among other things, establishment registration and product listing; donor eligibility; current good tissue practices covering all stages of cellular- and tissue-product production, including harvesting, processing, manufacture, storage, labeling, packaging, and distribution; and recommended controls intended to prevent the introduction, transmission, and spread of communicable diseases in humans.

For regulatory purposes, a processed HCT/P is not automatically treated as a drug product. Instead, a second distinction is made between drug and non-drug products on the basis of the totality of processing and manipulation (generally referred to as the minimal manipulation standard). Factors considered in making this distinction (and thus in the ultimate regulation of such products) include the degree of manipulation exerted on the product (ie, whether the product has been more than minimally manipulated), whether the product is intended for a homologous function, whether the product has been combined with noncellular or nontissue components, and the product's overall effect or dependence on the body's metabolic function.[8]

An HCT/P that falls short of the established minimal manipulation standard will be treated as a biologic, requiring its manufacturer to register its establishment, list the product with FDA, and adopt and implement procedures for the control of communicable diseases. An HCT/P exceeding the established standard, however, will be treated as a drug product requiring the filing of an investigational new drug application (IND) and the eventual review and approval of a new drug application (NDA) before marketing and sale.

An IND notifies the FDA of prospective clinical testing and allows the test product to be shipped in interstate commerce. Data collected during the IND is then used to support an NDA. Approval of an NDA requires a showing that the drug is safe and effective for its intended use and that the methods, facilities, and controls used for the manufacturing, processing, and packaging of the drug are adequate to preserve its identity, strength, quality, and purity. In the United States, the IND and NDA processes can be both time consuming and costly.

FDA's CURRENT AND POTENTIAL FUTURE REGULATION OF VETERINARY REGENERATIVE MEDICINE

All indications suggest that veterinary cellular- and tissue-based products (VCT/Ps) will be regulated under CVM's existing statutory and regulatory framework for veterinary drug products with heavy reliance on the HCT/P regulations as a guide. It is a near certainty that CVM will treat at least some veterinary HCT/P as drugs. Whether CVM will take a multifaceted regulatory approach as the FDA did on the human side, with a distinction being made between drugs and non-drugs for regulatory purposes, has yet to be determined.

Relying on an understanding of the HCT/Ps regulations as guidance, one would suspects (and hopes) that a distinction will be made between VCT/Ps on the basis of factors such as degree of manipulation, intended use, composition, and metabolic interaction. Like their human counterparts, those falling below a certain threshold would be treated as simply cells and tissues requiring only establishment registration and product listing, and safeguards to prevent the introduction, transmission, and spread of communicable diseases. Those exceeding the relevant adopted (ie, a hypothetical veterinary minimal manipulation standard), would be subjected to a greater degree of regulatory scrutiny and required to open an INADA, file an NADA, and obtain agency approval before marketing and sale. VCT/Ps involving rigorous culturing and processing of harvested cells and tissues would therefore likely be treated as drugs. We have already seen some concrete indications of FDA adopting such an approach. On June 30, 2011 Medistem Inc. announced that licensee and collaborator Renovo-Cyte LLC was assigned INAD numbers by FDA to study the use of endometrial regenerative cells (ERC) in dogs, cats, rabbits and horses.[a]

---

[a] See Medistem Licensee RenovoCyte LLC receives FDA INAD for universal donor endometrial regenerative cells (ERC); Medistem Press Release (June 30, 2011).

Applying this hypothetical regulatory structure to veterinary regenerative therapies, allogeneic-based products versus autologous treatments would likely be treated as drugs and subject to more rigorous regulatory scrutiny because of the greater perceived risk of contamination and disease transmission. Under such an approach, it is also possible that VCT/P using cells harvested from different parts of the body (ie, fat, bone marrow, cord blood), could be treated differently for regulatory purposes.

At the time of writing, there are several commercial regenerative therapies available in the market. To date, the FDA has generally taken a wait-and-see approach and has exercised enforcement discretion with regards to such products. Until specific regulations or guidelines are implemented, a VCT/P is approved, or the agency takes enforcement action, the FDA is likely to extend enforcement discretion regarding such products.

Parties interested in commercializing VCT/Ps should be actively monitoring and engaged in the regulatory development process. Because formal regulations and guidelines have yet to be adopted and implemented, and considering CVM's willingness to meet with the industry to understand the science and technology of regenerative medicine, this combination of circumstances creates a unique and valuable opportunity for the clinicians and the industry to be involved in the development process.

THE RISKS ASSOCIATED WITH MARKETING AND PROMOTING VETERINARY REGENERATIVE MEDICINE

Caution must be taken when marketing and promoting VCT/Ps in the United States, especially in the absence of FDA review and approval. Failure to properly substantiate a claim could result in a product being deemed adulterated or misbranded.

At the time of writing, there is no evidence to indicate that the FDA has taken enforcement action against the marketing and sale of any veterinary regenerative therapies or products specifically. However, we have already seen enforcement action against several individuals and firms involved in the marketing and sale of regenerative products for human use. In one such case, the agency has gone so far as to pursue court action. Just as the future regulation of veterinary regenerative medicine might be predicted from the FDA's approach to regulating HCT/Ps, it may also be possible to predict how the FDA will pursue enforcement action in the veterinary profession by reviewing its current enforcement in the human market.

All indications suggest that the FDA is taking a wait-and-see approach to enforcement while the industry evolves. Relying on history as a guide, however, as the industry grows and the FDA develops a greater understanding of the practice, the agency is likely to become more involved. This point will be particularly true as firms move forward with commercializing the practice for widespread use in the form of off-the-shelf products and as practitioners and firms become more aggressive in the marketing and promotion of their unapproved regenerative therapies and products.

All labeling and advertising must be truthful and not misleading. Under a Memorandum of Understanding between the FDA and the Federal Trade Commission (FTC), the FDA retains primary jurisdiction over labeling, whereas the FTC has primary regulatory jurisdiction over advertising. This article focuses exclusively on the FDA's regulation of labeling and promotional materials.

For regulatory purposes, the term labeling includes all marketing and promotional materials, including container and package labels, package inserts, shipping labels, Web sites, trade show flyers and posters, journal articles, and advertisements. As a general rule, all labeling and promotional claims must be adequately substantiated by competent and reliable scientific evidence.

The FDA uses a variety of methods, including facility inspections and general monitoring of the marketplace, to ensure compliance with its rules and regulations. When minor deficiencies are observed during an inspection, parties are frequently given an opportunity to voluntarily resolve them. For more significant violations, a warning letter might be issued. Where noncompliance poses a significant or immediate threat to the public health or where compliance is not achieved via a warning letter, the FDA might resort to more aggressive enforcement methods, such as product seizure or detention; recall; temporary or permanent injunction; debarment; civil penalties; and, in the most serious of cases, criminal proceedings, including prison.

A discussion of various types of marketing and promotional claims used by individuals and firms, and their potential risks, is included next. Afterwards, a summary of a current and ongoing FDA action involving the marketing and sale of a stem cell–based therapy for human use is provided.

Types of Labeling and Promotional Claims and Their Potential Risks

Various types of labeling and promotional claims, and examples of recent FDA enforcement actions associated with the use of such claims, are provided next.

Disease claims

A disease claim is a claim that addresses a product's ability to diagnose, cure, mitigate, treat, or prevent disease. Apart from limited exceptions, disease claims are not permitted to appear on a product's label or labeling unless the product and the claim have been reviewed and approved by the FDA.

In September 2008, the FDA issued a warning letter to a firm marketing and promoting various unapproved joint-related products as supplements for veterinary use. The firm claimed that the products could be used to treat various therapeutic conditions, including to "manage the crippling effects of osteoarthritis," "works by actually healing the damage that has been done," "builds cartilage," "reduces pain," and "treats arthritis in dogs." Citing the included disease claims, the FDA deemed the products unapproved new animal drugs for which required safety and efficacy had not been shown.[9]

Unsubstantiated efficacy claims

Companies and individuals must be able to substantiate that all labeling and advertising claims are truthful and not misleading. A general rule to mitigate the potential risk of enforcement action is to ensure that all claims are properly and adequately substantiated. In terms of defining what constitutes adequate substantiation, the FDA relies on a standard provided by the FTC. The FTC standard of competent and reliable scientific evidence has been defined in FTC case law as "tests, analyses, research, studies, or other evidence based on the expertise of professionals in the relevant area, that has been conducted and evaluated in an objective manner by persons qualified to do so, using procedures generally accepted in the profession to yield accurate and reliable results."[10] In cases where a product is deemed to be unsafe or lack efficacy, there is a considerable risk that the FDA could require a product to be removed from the market.

In June 2007, the CVM issued a warning letter to a major veterinary pharmaceutical manufacturer. The warning letter was issued in response to claims featured on the firm's Web site for an approved oral antiparasitic drug product indicated for the prevention of heartworm disease. The company's Web site contained unsubstantiated effectiveness claims suggesting that the product was also effective for the prevention, removal, or control of whipworms. Unaware of substantial evidence to support a claim of effectiveness against whipworms, the FDA requested that the company agree to immediately cease dissemination of the materials. The company agreed.[11]

Unsupported superiority claims

There are risks associated with the use of superiority claims. When making such claims, an individual or firm needs to maintain adequate substantiation on file in case the statements are questioned by the FDA or, more likely, by a competitor in the marketplace. In the absence of sufficient substantiation, claims will be considered false or misleading and render a product misbranded.

In September 2010, the FDA found that the manufacturer of an approved bovine product was making unsubstantiated superiority claims on its Web site. The claims suggested that the firm's cattle product was superior to those of its competitors, but the claims were not supported by substantial evidence or substantial clinical experience. In a letter to the firm, the FDA said that it was unaware of peer-reviewed, head-to-head studies demonstrating the superiority of the subject product over other similarly situated products on the market.[12]

Consumer testimonials

Consumer experience is not a legitimate basis for claims that are not otherwise sufficiently substantiated. The use of consumer testimonials poses a significant risk to the marketers of a veterinary product where such statements are misleading, unsubstantiated, and improperly imply effectiveness. If included on a firm's Web site or within its marketing materials, a testimonial is considered labeling and can be used to determine a product's intended use. The FTC has stated that advertisers may not use endorsements or testimonials with representations that would be deceptive or not substantiated if made directly by the advertiser.[13] For this reason, it is generally recommended that individuals and firms avoid using consumer testimonials in their marketing and promotion.

In a June 2009 warning letter, the FDA alleged that the recipient was marketing and selling an unapproved veterinary drug product for the treatment of arthritis and other joint conditions. The product was deemed misbranded on the basis of, among other things, a consumer's testimonial and praise for the product on the product Web site: "My dog was hit by a car several years ago, and unfortunately lost a lot of his ability to move around. Just a couple of weeks after trying this product, he was actually running. I couldn't believe it!" Citing that testimonial and other unsubstantiated statements, the FDA determined that the product was not safe and effective for use under the conditions prescribed, recommended, or suggested in the labeling.[14]

FDA Enforcement Action Involving Stem Cell Therapies for Human Use

The FDA has taken enforcement action against several individuals and firms for the marketing and promotion of unapproved stem cell–based therapies for human use. In each case, the products were deemed adulterated or misbranded on the basis of failure to obtain an approved NDA, failure to comply with the agency's relevant regulations (ie, current good manufacturing practices), the use of unsubstantiated labeling or promotional claims, or some combination of all of these factors. Although multiple enforcement actions have been taken, this section focuses exclusively on a case involving the FDA and Regenerative Services.

The argument over FDA regulation versus the practice of medicine

The case of the *FDA v Regenerative Services, LLC* (RS)[15] focuses on the marketing and sale of stem cell–based therapies in the United States, and addresses the question of whether such therapies constitute an FDA-regulated drug product or simply the professional practice of medicine. The case is currently ongoing and the eventual outcome will certainly have an impact on the regulation of regenerative medicine for both human and veterinary use.

The FDA sent RS a letter in July 2008 questioning the regulatory status of its promoted products. By way of background, RS was marketing and promoting a cultured stem cell–based treatment for the regeneration of bone and cartilage in humans suffering from painful orthopedic conditions. The promoted therapy involved the harvesting of mesenchymal stem cells from a patient's bone marrow, the isolation and subsequent growth of the cells using growth factors drawn from the patient's blood, and the reinjection of the cells back into the patient's own body.[16]

To market and promote their offered services, RS used treatment claims and consumer testimonials on its Web site. RS claimed that the promoted procedure "relieves pain and restores mobility and is a safer, less disruptive alternative to surgery… [and] almost anyone with joint pain or non-healing fractures can benefit from this ground-breaking procedure." As for consumer testimonials, the Web site included a statement from an alleged RS patient stating, "I dealt with knee pain and the problems for a long time, … I would absolutely recommend that anybody with osteoarthritis check out [the procedures and] … I want the whole world – especially seniors – to know that injuries such as femoral, hip and pelvic fractures don't have to diminish your quality of life."

Citing the included claims and testimonials, among other violations, the FDA deemed the offered therapy to be an unapproved new drug intended for use in the diagnosis, cure, mitigation, treatment, or prevention of disease in man for which FDA approval had not been obtained. The FDA also found the offered therapy to be adulterated based on the fact that the used cells exceeded the minimal manipulation standard because they were being used for nonhomologous uses.

Prompted by the July 2008 letter and a series of later events, RS sued the FDA in February 2009 seeking declaratory and injunctive relief from the FDA's regulation. RS argued that the offered therapy constituted the practice of medicine, which falls outside the FDA's regulatory jurisdiction. The FDA counterargued that, although it may not directly interfere with a physician's prescribing habits, it may limit what drugs are available to physicians to prescribe in the US market. The case was dismissed by the court in February 2009 as premature.

RS refiled the case in June 2010 after the FDA conducted another inspection of the RS facility identifying several additional deficiencies. In court documents, RS again argued that the promoted therapy constituted the practice of medicine. It also challenged the FDA's definition of minimal manipulation as arbitrary and capricious, claiming that the public should have been provided with an opportunity for notice and comment. In response, the FDA filed a countersuit in August 2010 seeking to permanently enjoin RS from using stem cells to treat patients without first obtaining FDA drug approval.

In January 2011, the US Department of Justice (DOJ), on behalf of the FDA, filed a motion for summary judgment and a motion to dismiss RS's counterclaims. DOJ argued that there is no issue of material fact in the case because RS is clearly manufacturing, marketing, and selling an unapproved new drug product in interstate commerce in violation of the FDCA and the regulations. It likewise argued that the unapproved drug is also adulterated on the basis of RS's failure to comply with the agency's applicable regulations and that the promoted therapy is misbranded because of RS's use of several unsubstantiated labeling and promotional claims.

The initial July 2008 letter to RS was important from an industry perspective because it provided one of the earliest and most detailed impressions of how the FDA was interpreting the HCT/P regulations. It generally confirmed the industry assumption that the FDA would pursue a 2-prong regulatory pathway for HCT/Ps, with a distinction being made on the basis of the amount of manipulation or processing. As for the ongoing case, it remains critically important to the industry because of the general policy questions it raises regarding the use of HCT/Ps therapy in humans. Among other things, the court's decision in the case should expand on the industry's understanding of the parameters of the professional practice of medicine exception and further interpret the FDA's authority to regulate therapeutic products in that practice. A decision could be issued later this year.

SUMMARY

As extrapolated from the FDA's regulation of regenerative medicine and its related products for human use, it is reasonable to assume that the FDA will assert regulatory jurisdiction over the marketing and sale of those veterinary therapies and products offered for commercial use. Although specific rules and regulations pertaining to veterinary regenerative medicine have yet to be proposed and adopted by the FDA, it is safe for the industry to anticipate the FDA requiring drug review and approval for at least some promoted products, especially those exceeding the referenced minimal manipulation standard. If a serious issue arises (ie, similar to the death of the 21 polo ponies in Florida in April 2009) or a significant threat to the public well-being is identified, FDA regulation will probably be adopted sooner rather than later. For the time being, however, the FDA appears to be exercising enforcement discretion with regard to the practice on a general industry-wide scale. Although this does not prevent the FDA from taking regulatory enforcement action against persons or firms improperly harvesting, processing, storing, labeling, and promoting their products, its does lessen the overall immediate risk. By working to ensure compliance with the FDA's applicable statutory and regulatory provisions and by avoiding the use of unsubstantiated disease and superiority claims, consumer testimonials, and other false and misleading promotional materials, individuals and firms can further mitigate the limited enforcement risk that currently exists in the market.

REFERENCES

1. FDCA Section 201(v).
2. FDCA Section 512.
3. FDA and the Veterinarian, Glossary; October 28, 2009. Accessed July 25, 2011.
4. Also 21 USC §§151–158; United States v Miami Serpentarium Laboratories, Inc, Food, Drug, Cosm L. Rep. (CCH); 1982–83. Dev. Trans. Binder 38, 164 (S.D. Fla. 1982).
5. Animal & Veterinary: A Brief Overview of CVM's Drug Approval Process, FDA and the Veterinarian; FDA Guidance Document; December 14, 2009. Accessed July 25, 2011.
6. 21 C.F.R. Part 1271.
7. 21 C.F.R. § 1271.3(d).
8. 21 C.F.R. § 1271.10.
9. FDA Warning Letter, MIN 08-17; September 5, 2008. Accessed July 25, 2011.
10. Vital Basics, Inc, C-4107 (Consent April 26, 2004); see also In Re Schering Corp, 118 FTC 1030, 1123; 1994.
11. Stamps C. CVM has significant role in regulating advertising labeling of new animal drug, FDA Veterinarian Newsletter, CVM Publication; Vol. XXIII, No. 1; 2008.
12. FDA Action Letter, NADA 113–645; September 16, 2010.
13. 16 C.F.R. § 255.1(a).
14. FDA Warning Letter, WIL 17-09; June 2, 2009.
15. FDA v Regenerative Services, LLC.
16. FDA Untitled Letter to Regenerative Services, Inc; July 25, 2008.

Cell-based Therapies: Current Issues and Future Directions

Matthew C. Stewart, BVSc, MVetClinStud, PhD

KEYWORDS

• Mesenchymal stem cells • Biologics • Efficacy • Clinical trials

It is clear from the information presented in the preceding articles that the ongoing development of cell-based and related biologic therapies promises a great deal for both medical and veterinary clinicians, particularly in conditions in which the resultant scar-based repair or underlying degenerative nature of the disease prevents functional recovery. Equine veterinarians have been, and remain, at the forefront of these developments, particularly regarding orthopedic applications. However, as eloquently stated by Dr Wes Sutter in a recent review article,

> ... the availability of these (cell-based) therapies to the equine practitioner has out-paced needed experimental and clinical data necessary to establish efficacy and safety.[1]

Accepting the current optimism regarding cell-based therapies, there are still many aspects of these treatments, and related biologics, that need to be clarified.

HORSES FOR COURSES? SOURCES, DOSES, AND TIMING

In reference to Dr Sutter's statement above, the current sources of stem cells for equine applications are largely based on ease of collection, and both the doses of mesenchymal stem cells (MSCs) and timing of administration are determined by variable combinations of educated guesswork and the logistics of case presentation.[1] As an informative example, although the area adjacent to the tail head is commonly used for adipose tissue collection in the horse, because of ease of access and cosmetic issues, there is compelling evidence that the specific stem cell properties of fat-derived cells vary considerably with anatomic location. Adipose-derived MSCs isolated from intraarticular fat depots are substantially more chondrogenic than MSCs derived from nonarticular adipose sites.[2,3] Similarly, MSCs derived from synovium have greater chondrogenic potential than MSCs derived from other sources.[4,5] Future

---

The author has nothing to disclose.
Department of Veterinary Clinical Medicine, College of Veterinary Medicine, University of Illinois, 1008 West Hazelwood Drive, Urbana, IL 61802, USA
E-mail address: matt1@illinois.edu

Vet Clin Equine 27 (2011) 393–399
doi:10.1016/j.cveq.2011.07.001
0749-0739/11/$ – see front matter © 2011 Elsevier Inc. All rights reserved.

investigations should determine whether MSCs isolated from different tissues and anatomic locations exhibit biologic activities that provide advantages for specific clinical applications, independent of the expediencies associated with collection protocols. As another example, there is a general agreement that MSCs injected into acutely traumatized and inflamed tissues will fare badly; however, it is also possible that the antiinflammatory and neoangiogenic activities of MSCs might positively influence the early phases of repair and affect long-term benefits. Conversely, there is presumably a point in the postinjury healing process in which the abilities of stem cells to influence inflammation and fibrosis and participate in tissue regeneration are missed; yet this window of opportunity has not been well defined. These questions can only be answered by appropriately designed and controlled studies and will likely require a repeatable injury model for initial experiments, with corroboration of the findings through clinical case management.

HOMEGROWN OR OFF-THE-SHELF? AUTOLOGOUS VERSUS ALLOGENEIC STEM CELLS

At present, most clinical studies and in-practice protocols are based on autologous MSC administration, whereby cells are collected from, and then delivered back to, the same patient. Autologous MSC collection is a straightforward process (covered in detail by Taylor and Clegg in this issue) but requires some specialized equipment and facilities and can take a few minutes for minimally altered aspirates to several weeks for in vitro expansion of MSC cultures. If expanded autologous MSC populations are needed, the mandatory delay until the cells are available for administration can be prohibitive.

The facts that stem cells lack major histocompatibility complex II antigens[6] and are able to avoid immune recognition[7,8] allow for allogeneic administration of these cells. In effect, MSC and embryonic stem cell (ESC) cultures can be established from suitable donors to generate off-the-shelf allogeneic cell stocks for immediate administration. This possibility will be necessary for ESC applications, because these cells need to be generated from the inner cell mass of equine blastocysts, as detailed by Hackett and Fortier elsewhere in this issue. There are several nominal advantages associated with ESC technologies. First, these cells can be maintained in vitro as cell lines with essentially unlimited proliferative capacity, provided appropriate culture conditions are maintained. Second, ESCs are capable of differentiating into all adult tissue lineages, with the potential to affect a wide range of pathologic conditions. Preliminary in vivo studies in horses have shown that ESCs persist at sites of intratendinous injection longer than MSCs[9] and improve tendon healing in the collagenase-induced superficial digital flexor tendon (SDFT) tendinitis model.[10] There was no evidence of a host immune response to implanted ESCs in either study, nor was there any indication of teratoma formation, but these studies were both short term (90 and 56 days, respectively); tumor development after ESC administration remains a distinct possibility (in vivo teratoma formation is one of the cardinal assays for ESC identity) and will require much longer study intervals before ESCs can be considered safe for clinical use. It is almost certain that the Federal regulatory authorities will classify allogeneic MSC and ESC preparations as drugs that require proof of both safety and efficacy for approval (as discussed in this issue by Nobert). These demonstrations will undoubtedly be challenging to organize and expensive to execute.

ARE STEM CELLS REALLY NECESSARY?

Although much of the attention on cell-based therapies has been focused on the processing and application of comparatively pure stem cell populations, this is currently a prolonged and tedious process, requiring several weeks of in vitro culturing. As discussed in this issue by Stewart and Stewart and also by Taylor and Clegg, immunophenotyping of equine stem cells is still poorly characterized, and establishing a reliable protocol for fluorescence-activated cell sorter–based equine MSC isolation will require considerable investment in antibody generation and epitope validation.[6] In addition, immunophenotypically similar stem cell populations can exhibit different biologic activities,[11–13] and there are no compelling clinical data indicating any intrinsic superiority of purified MSC populations over more heterogeneous cell isolates for orthopedic applications.

Accepting the issues raised in the previous paragraph, there is an increasing body of evidence that purified stem cell populations are not necessary for effective biologic therapy. As detailed by Stewart and Stewart, bone marrow aspirate concentrate (BMAC) has been used effectively to stimulate bone repair in human patients[14–16] and improve articular cartilage resurfacing and tendon repair in horses.[17,18] Adipose-derived stromal vascular fraction (ADSVF), the cellular product derived from fat digestion and marketed by Vet-Stem (Poway, CA, USA), has been used successfully in the equine collagenase-induced SDFT tendinitis model[19] and in many clinical cases.[1] Impressive clinical responses have been reported after administration of platelet-rich plasma (PRP) and autologous-conditioned serum (ACS) for tendon/ligament injuries[20,21] and osteoarthritis,[22] respectively (covered in detail by Textor elsewhere in this issue).

Given these clinically significant results, along with the obvious convenience and cost-effectiveness derived from point-of-service collection and administration, biologics such as PRP, ACS, BMAC, and ADSVF may well make stem cell therapy obsolete before it becomes established as a mainstream therapy in equine practice. Direct clinical comparisons in matched clinical cases and experimental lesion model–based studies will be needed to address this possibility but, from a clinical perspective, functional recovery is a more important goal than authentic tissue regeneration per se.

The need for exogenous MSC administration could also be avoided by recruiting clinically effective numbers of host MSCs to injury sites. MSCs are stimulated to enter the systemic circulation and migrate to sites of injury in response to chemotactic cues, a process referred to as homing. The perivascular location of most MSC niches facilitates this mobilization. A range of growth factors, inflammatory cytokines, and chemokines regulate stem cell migration and homing.[23,24] The best characterized is the chemokine stromal-derived factor 1 that binds to C-X-C chemokine receptor type 4 on the cell surface of target stem cells.[25,26] Although the intrinsic mechanisms in place to recruit stem cells to sites of injury are self-evidently inadequate (otherwise, everything would heal spontaneously without the need for intervention), delivery of key chemokines and/or growth factors to sites of injury could be used to attract and retain sufficient MSC numbers for effective repair. This approach complements tissue engineering strategies for tissue regeneration; chemokines could be incorporated into bioinformative scaffolds to attract and then regulate host stem cells at the site of implantation.

MSCs, NOT JUST AN ORTHOPEDIC RESOURCE

The multilineage potential of MSCs has resulted in a great deal of attention being focused on the tissue regenerative applications of these cells for cartilage, bone, and tendon/ligament repair. However, as the understanding of stem cell biology increases, it is now clear that MSCs represent effective therapeutic agents for a range of disease conditions. In particular, the immunomodulatory activities of MSCs have been applied in people for the treatment of several immune-driven diseases, such as multiple sclerosis, graft-versus-host disease, solid organ transplantation, and

Crohn disease.[27–30] A large number of experimental studies using rodent models support the use of MSC therapy for rheumatoid arthritis and related conditions.[31] Stem cells also have the potential to resolve select genetically based diseases, such as osteogenesis imperfecta,[32] in which a genetically dysfunctional cell population can be replaced by genetically normal stem cells through host cell depletion and subsequent stem cell engraftment.

Immune-mediated, autoimmune, and genetic diseases are not common in the equine population. However, at recent veterinary conferences focused on regenerative medicine and stem cell therapies, there have been informal discussions describing stem cell therapy for the treatment of laminitis, exercise-induced pulmonary hemorrhage, lower airway disease, and wound repair and as an adjunct therapy for spinal cord disease (Douglas Herthel and Eric Carlson, personal communications, 2011). Given the broad range of MSC trophic activities and their capacities to stimulate neoangiogenesis, reduce inflammation, recruit host progenitor cells, and minimize fibrosis (as discussed in this issue by Stewart and Stewart and also by Peroni and Borjesson), the conceptual bases for stem cell administration for these conditions are clear. Undoubtedly, new applications for cell-based therapies will be recognized as the understanding of stem cell biology increases.

OF COURSE, STEM CELLS WORK! DEMONSTRATING EFFICACY

As noted by Dr Sutter and Clegg and Pinchbeck of this issue, the widespread use of stem cells in equine practice is not currently supported by rigorous experimental and clinical data. In fact, some experimental studies have shown little or no benefit after intraarticular MSC administration for the treatment of arthritis or cartilage repair in horses,[33,34] and although several reports that used the collagenase-induced SDFT lesion model have shown improved repair tissue organization at the histologic level,[10,35–37] no return-to-function outcome measures were included in these analyses.

Credible demonstration of efficacy for cell-based therapies should be a collective goal of the equine veterinary community from an ethical perspective, but it may well become mandatory if the Food and Drug Administration decides that some or all cell-based therapies will require convincing data supporting safety and efficacy before approval. This issue is addressed in detail in the article by Nobert. Clinical trials to assess efficacy of any given cell-based therapy certainly require multi-institutional practice, participation, and coordination, as has been established for previous assessments of β-aminopropionitrile for SDFT strain injuries, tiludronate for navicular disease, and, most recently, the value of MSCs for equine arthritis, organized by investigators at the Colorado State University.[38] To put this in perspective, the clinical trials that led to the approval of recombinant bone morphogenetic protein 2 for the treatment of tibial fractures,[39] tibial nonunions,[40] and spinal fusion[41] in human patients required the recruitment of 450, 122, and 279 patients, respectively. Given the interpatient and patient management variables that undoubtedly exist in any clinical study of cell-based therapy for equine flexor tendinitis, osteoarthritis, suspensory desmitis, or other candidate condition, similar case numbers will be required to generate sufficient statistical power.

In addition to adequate subject recruitment, a consistent and standardized panel of objective outcome measures will need to be developed to rigorously assess clinical outcome. Magnetic resonance imaging, radiology, and ultrasonography provide noninvasive imaging modalities that can plausibly assess reparative responses in tendon, ligament, bone, and articular lesions, whereas force plate and gait analysis measurements can provide quantitative indices of functional recovery to corroborate clinicians' assessments and return-to-competition results.

Accepting the significant challenges outlined previously, cell-based therapies provide equine practitioners with feasible options for the treatment of common musculoskeletal conditions in performance horses that have no reliably effective treatment at present.

REFERENCES

1. Sutter WW. Therapy for tendon and ligament injuries. Clin Tech Equine Pract 2007;6:198–208.
2. Mochizuki T, Muneta T, Sakaguchi Y, et al. Higher chondrogenic potential of fibrous synovium– and adipose synovium–derived cells compared with subcutaneous fat–derived cells. Arthritis Rheum 2006;54:843–53.
3. English A, Jones EA, Corscadden D, et al. A comparative assessment of cartilage and joint fat pad as a potential source of cells for autologous therapy development in knee osteoarthritis. Rheumatology 2007;46:1676–83.
4. Sakaguchi Y, Sekiya I, Yagishita K, et al. Comparison of human stem cells derived from various mesenchymal tissues. Arthritis Rheum 2005;52:2521–9.
5. Yoshimura H, Muneta T, Nimura A, et al. Comparison of rat mesenchymal stem cells derived from bone marrow, synovium, periosteum, adipose tissue, and muscle. Cell Tissue Res 2007;327:449–62.
6. De Schauwer C, Meyer E, Van de Walle GR, et al. Markers of stemness in equine mesenchymal stem cells: a plea for uniformity. Theriogenology 2010; 75:1431–43.
7. Tse WT, Pendleton JD, Beyer WM, et al. Suppression of allogeneic T-cell proliferation by human marrow stromal cells: implications in transplantation. Transplantation 2003;75:389–97.
8. Aggarwal S, Pittenger MF. Human mesenchymal stem cells modulate allogeneic immune cell responses. Blood 2005;105:1815–22.
9. Guest DJ, Smith MR, Allen WR. Equine embryonic stem-like cells and mesenchymal stromal cells have different survival rates and migration patterns following their injection into damaged superficial digital flexor tendon. Equine Vet J 2010; 42:636–42.
10. Watts AE, Yeager AE, Kopyov OV, et al. Fetal derived embryonic-like stem cells improve healing in a large animal flexor tendonitis model. Stem Cell Res Ther 2011;2:4.
11. Im G, Shin Y, Lee K. Do adipose tissue-derived mesenchymal stem cells have the same osteogenic and chondrogenic potential as bone marrow-derived cells? Osteoarthritis Cartilage 2005;13:845–53.
12. Rebelatto CK, Aguiar AM, Moretao MP, et al. Dissimilar differentiation of mesenchymal stem cells from bone marrow, umbilical cord blood, and adipose tissue. Exp Biol Med 2008;233:901–13.
13. Danišovic L, Varga I, Polak S, et al. Comparison of in vitro chondrogenic potential of human mesenchymal stem cells derived from bone marrow and adipose tissue. Gen Physiol Biophys 2009;28:56–62.
14. Jäger M, Herten M, Fochtmann U, et al. Bridging the gap: bone marrow aspiration concentrate reduces autologous bone grafting in osseous defects. J Orthop Res 2010;29:173–80.
15. Hernigou P, Poignard A, Beaujean F, et al. Percutaneous autologous bone-marrow grafting for nonunions: influence of the number and concentration of progenitor cells. J Bone Joint Surg Am 2005;87:1430–7.

16. Vadalá G, Di Martino A, Tirindelli MC, et al. Use of autologous bone marrow cells concentrate enriched with platelet-rich fibrin on corticocancellous bone allograft for posterolateral multilevel cervical fusion. J Tissue Eng Regen Med 2008;2:515–20.

17. Crovace A, Lacitignola L, Rossi G, et al. Histological and immunohistochemical evaluation of autologous cultured bone marrow mesenchymal stem cells and bone marrow mononucleated cells in collagenase-induced tendinitis of equine superficial digital flexor tendon. Vet Med Int 2010;2010:250978.

18. Fortier LA, Potter HG, Rickey EJ, et al. Concentrated bone marrow aspirate improves full-thickness cartilage repair compared with microfracture in the equine model. J Bone Joint Surg Am 2010;92:1927–37.

19. Nixon AJ, Dahlgren LA, Haupt JL, et al. Effect of adipose-derived nucleated cell fractions on tendon repair in horses with collagenase-induced tendinitis. Am J Vet Res 2008;69:928–37.

20. Waselau M, Sutter WW, Genovese RL, et al. Intralesional injection of platelet-rich plasma followed by controlled exercise for treatment of midbody suspensory ligament desmitis in Standardbred racehorses. J Am Vet Med Assoc 2008;232: 1515–20.

21. Bosch G, van Schie HT, de Groot MW, et al. Effects of platelet-rich plasma on the quality of repair of mechanically induced core lesions in equine superficial digital flexor tendons: a placebo-controlled experimental study. J Orthop Res 2010;28: 211–7.

22. Frisbie DD, Kawcak CE, Werpy NM, et al. Clinical, biochemical, and histologic effects of intra-articular administration of autologous conditioned serum in horses with experimentally induced osteoarthritis. Am J Vet Res 2007;68:290–6.

23. Ozaki Y, Nishimura M, Sekiya K, et al. Comprehensive analysis of chemotactic factors for bone marrow mesenchymal stem cells. Stem Cell Dev 2007;16: 119–29.

24. Ponte AL, Marais E, Gallay N, et al. Mesenchymal stem cells: comparison of chemokine and growth factor chemotactic activities. Stem Cells 2007;25:1737–45.

25. Bhaktaa S, Hong P, Koc O, et al. The surface adhesion molecule CXCR4 stimulates mesenchymal stem cell migration to stromal cell-derived factor-1 in vitro but does not decrease apoptosis under serum deprivation. Cardiovasc Revasc Med 2006;7:19–24.

26. Ji JF, He BP, Dheen ST, et al. Interactions of chemokines and chemokine receptors mediate the migration of stem cells to the impaired site in the brain after hypoglossal nerve injury. Stem Cells 2004;22:415–27.

27. Le Blanc K, Frassoni F, Ball L, et al. Mesenchymal stem cells for treatment of steroid-resistant, severe, acute graft-versus-host disease: a phase II study. Lancet 2008;371:1579–86.

28. Freedman MS, Bar-Or A, Atkins HL, et al. The therapeutic potential of mesenchymal stem cell transplantation as a treatment for multiple sclerosis: consensus report of the International MSCT Study Group. Mult Scler 2010;16:503–10.

29. Hoogduijn MJ, Popp FC, Grohnert A, et al. Advancement of mesenchymal stem cell therapy in solid organ transplantation (MISOT). Transplantation 2010;90: 124–6.

30. Shi Y, Hu G, Su J, et al. Mesenchymal stem cells: a new strategy for immunosuppression and tissue repair. Cell Res 2010;20:510–8.

31. Djouad F, Bouffi C, Ghannam S, et al. Mesenchymal stem cells: innovative therapeutic tools for rheumatic diseases. Nat Rev Rheumatol 2009;5:392–9.

32. Horwitz EM, Prockop DJ, Gordon PL, et al. Clinical responses to bone marrow transplantation in children with severe osteogenesis imperfecta. Blood 2001;97: 1227–31.

33. Wilke MM, Nydam DV, Nixon AJ. Enhanced early chondrogenesis in articular defects following arthroscopic mesenchymal stem cell implantation in an equine model. J Orthop Res 2007;25:913–25.

34. Frisbie DD, Kisiday JD, Kawcak CE, et al. Evaluation of adipose derived stromal vascular fraction or bone marrow derived mesenchymal stem cells for treatment of osteoarthritis. J Orthop Res 2009;27:1675–80.

35. Crovace A, Lacitignola L, De Siena R, et al. Cell therapy for tendon repair in horses: an experimental study. Vet Res Commun 2007;31(Suppl 1):281–3.

36. Schnabel LV, Lynch ME, van der Meulen MC, et al. Mesenchymal stem cells and insulin-like growth factor-I gene-enhanced mesenchymal stem cells improve structural aspects of healing in equine flexor digitorum superficialis tendons. J Orthop Res 2009;27:1392–8.

37. Carvalho A, Alves A, de Oliveira P, et al. Use of adipose tissue-derived mesenchymal stem cells for experimental tendinitis therapy in equines. J Equine Vet Sci 2011;31:26–34.

38. Ferris DJ, Frisbie DD, Kisiday JD, et al. Clinical follow-up of horses treated with bone marrow derived mesenchymal stem cells for musculoskeletal lesions. Proc AAEP Ann Conv 2009;55:59.

39. Govender S, Csimma C, Genant HK, et al. Recombinant human bone morphogenetic protein-2 for treatment of open tibial fractures: a prospective, controlled, randomized study of four hundred and fifty patients. J Bone Joint Surg Am 2002;84:2123–34.

40. Friedlaender GE, Perry CR, Cole JD, et al. Osteogenic protein-1 (bone morphogenetic protein-7) in the treatment of tibial nonunions. J Bone Joint Surg Am 2001; 83(Suppl 1):S151–8.

41. Burkus JK, Gornet MF, Dickman CA, et al. Anterior lumbar interbody fusion using rhBMP-2 with tapered interbody cages. J Spinal Disord Tech 2002;15:337–49.

Index

Note: Page numbers of article titles are in **boldface** type.

A

Adipose tissue
  as source of MSCs, 248–249
Adipose tissue–derived stromal vascular fraction cells (ADSVFCs)
  for musculoskeletal injuries, 367–368
ADSVFCs. *See* Adipose tissue–derived stromal vascular fraction cells (ADSVFCs)
Advanced Regenerative Therapies, 365
Allogeneic stem cells
  autologous stem cells *vs.*, 394
Autologous stem cells
  allogeneic stem cells *vs.*, 394

B

B lymphocytes
  MSCs effects on, 356
Biomaterials
  in bone repair, 305–306
Bone grafts
  in bone repair, 303
Bone healing
  stem cells in
    noninvasive assessment of, 308–309
Bone marrow
  as source of MSCs, 248
Bone marrow aspirate, 325
Bone marrow aspirate concentrate
  for musculoskeletal injuries, 366–367
Bone repair
  site of
    osteogenesis at, 299–302
  stem cell–based therapies for, **299–314**
    bone grafts, 303
    described, 302
    EPCs, 305
    gene therapy–type, 306–307
    MSCs
      direct application of, 303–305
    osteoprogenitor cells
      periosteum as source of, 307
    scaffolds and biomaterials in, 305–306

Vet Clin Equine 27 (2011) 401–409
doi:10.1016/S0749-0739(11)00041-1
0749-0739/11/$ – see front matter © 2011 Elsevier Inc. All rights reserved.

vetequine.theclinics.com

Printed and bound by CPI Group (UK) Ltd, Croydon, CR0 4YY

03/10/2024

01040444-0014